The COMMONSENSE GUIDE to

Barbara Caleen Hansen, Ph.D.

Shauna S. Roberts, Ph.D.

Weight Loss

For People with Diabetes

New Mexico Diabetes
Library Project

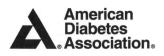
American Diabetes Association

BOOK ACQUISITIONS
Robert J. Anthony

EDITOR
Aime M. Ballard

PRODUCTION DIRECTOR
Carolyn R. Segree

PRODUCTION COORDINATOR
Peggy M. Rote

DESKTOP PUBLISHING
Harlowe Typography, Inc.

COVER DESIGN
Wickham & Associates, Inc.

Library of Congress Cataloging-in-Publication Data

Hansen, Barbara C.
 The common sense guide to weight loss for people with diabetes: how to lose weight—and keep it off—using medically proven techniques from the weight-loss experts/Barbara Hansen, and Shauna S. Roberts.
  p. cm.
  Includes index.
  ISBN 0-945448-85-6 (pbk.)
  1. Diabetes—Diet therapy. 2. Reducing diets. 3. Weight loss.
I. Roberts, Shauna S., 1956- . II. Title.
RC662.H37 1998
616.4'620654—DC21   97-45833
                           CIP

American Diabetes Association
1660 Duke Street, Alexandria, Virginia 22314

Printed in Canada
 3 5 7 9 10 8 6 4 2

Dedication

To David Scott Hansen, who confidently looks forward to a cure for diabetes.

—BCH

To the memory of Janet Louise Roberts.

—SSR

Contents

KEY

YOUR WEIGHT-LOSS PROGRAM MUST COORDINATE WITH YOUR DIABETES CARE

KEY

PERMANENT WEIGHT LOSS REQUIRES THAT YOU CHANGE YOUR LIFESTYLE FOR GOOD

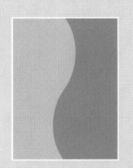

Acknowledgments

We are deeply grateful to the people who made this book possible:

- The people who generously shared their stories of weight-loss triumphs and failures and allowed us to use them in this book

- Ruth Bear and Marie McCarren, who helped us find the people whose stories we used

- Angela Lorio, who collected the stories

- Lauren Oddo, who transcribed tapes

- J. Shea Dixon, who provided legal and professional advice

- Those who supported us during the research and writing, including Noni L. Bodkin, Heidi K. Ortmeyer, and Maryne C. Glowacki

- Reynold and Dorothy Caleen, who provided the initial encouragement to develop this book

- All the health professionals and researchers who provided helpful reviews and suggestions, with special thanks to Deborah Riebe, Michael Weintraub, George A. Bray, George L. Blackburn, and Richard L. Atkinson

- Our husbands, Kenneth D. Hansen and David A. Malueg, and families, especially David S. Hansen, who encouraged us

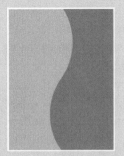

Introduction:
Why Do People With
Diabetes Need Their Own
Weight-Loss Book?

Maybe your doctor told you that losing weight is a big part of the treatment for your type 2 diabetes.

Or maybe you've been struggling with a weight problem for some time, and now you find out you have diabetes.

Or maybe your waistbands are getting a little tight, and you just happen to have diabetes.

Whatever your story, this book is for you if:

- You're an adult.

- You have some form of diabetes.

- You suspect you may be overweight or your doctor has told you that you are.

Like many aspects of life with diabetes, losing weight takes extra effort and thought. Everywhere you turn, magazines, TV, books, and your friends bombard you with advice on how to lose weight. But these sources leave plenty of questions unanswered for people with diabetes. How will losing weight affect your insulin or diabetes pill dose? Within your diabetes meal plan, how can you best cut back on calories? Can you exercise safely? How much exercise should someone with diabetes do? Can people with diabetes use weight-loss drugs?

Cutting through this tangle of questions is one reason this book exists. Another reason is that because you have diabetes, you need information about weight and fitness even more than other people do.

For people with type 2 diabetes, losing weight and exercising can greatly improve diabetes control. They may be able to lower their doses of diabetes pills or insulin—or even stop taking diabetes drugs altogether.

Eating right is a vital part of treatment for people with type 1 diabetes, too. In the past, people with type 1 diabetes usually didn't need to worry about being overweight. Poor glucose control often meant that they weighed too little, not too much. Today, many people with type 1 diabetes are working hard to keep their glucose levels as close to normal as possible. So they are no longer half-starved from poor control. But the same genes, fatty diet, and inactive lifestyle that lead to overweight among many Americans can now lead to overweight among people with type 1 diabetes.

In this book, you'll learn the seven crucial elements of weight loss for people with diabetes. These keys share a common theme: You can improve your life by improving your health. This book will help you to:

- Find a healthy weight and stay there, slashing your chances of getting serious diseases tied to excess weight

- Stay healthy longer

- Improve your glucose control and so slow or prevent diabetes complications

- Live life the way you deserve to—with joy and zest and verve!

Choosing the Right Target Weight Can Make the Difference Between Success and Failure.

You've decided it's time to make a change in your life. Congratulations! Choosing to lose weight can be the first step toward a happier, healthier life with fewer diabetes complications.

The first key to weight loss is that you need to figure out where you are and where you want to be. Research reveals that a broad range of weights can be healthful for people of a certain height. Despite what TV shows and ads tell you, a healthy weight does not mean being thin as a model. These chapters will help you choose a practical, healthy weight target based on your own circumstances.

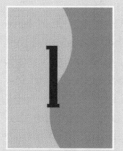

1

What a Healthy Weight Is—and Isn't

A healthy weight has little to do with beauty and everything to do with having a strong, healthy body that can live life to its fullest.

Losing weight is a lot like going on a trip. You probably wouldn't just jump in the car and head for the highway with no destination in mind. Rather, first you'd choose where you wanted to go. Then you'd choose a route. Probably you'd pick one that fit into your timetable for your trip, one that seemed practical and safe, yet would be enjoyable along the way.

The same plan works well when you start a weight-loss program. First, you should know where you are and decide where you're heading. Then you should choose a route.

That's where this book comes in. We'll talk about routes to weight loss later. But first, we'll help you decide where you are. Are you overweight? If so, how much? What do you hope to gain if you lose weight? How much weight is it practical for you to try to lose? These are important questions to answer before doing anything else.

HEALTHY WEIGHTS FOR ADULTS

You may already have some idea of what you want to weigh or think you should weigh. This weight may be based on what you weighed in college or at a time you felt and looked your best. It may be based on an actor you admire. Or it may be what your friends tell you you should weigh.

Science, too, has an opinion about your weight. Many scientists have studied disease rates in people of various weights. They have found that being heavier puts you at risk for many diseases. As a result of this research, charts and tables exist that can tell you what the healthiest weight range is for someone your height.

Because not all studies have found precisely the same cutoff for disease risk, not all weight tables agree with each other. And even if they did, being one place or another in a table is no guarantee of illness or health. Some overweight people live a long time with few health problems. Other people get heart disease or diabetes despite being at a good weight. These tables just give you an idea of the weight ranges that seem to be healthiest for the average person.

The Official, Government-Issue Weight Chart

Every few years, the U.S. Department of Agriculture and the U.S. Department of Health and Human Services ask experts to review the evidence on the relations among weight, diet, and health. The Departments then issue guidelines for eating a good diet. These guidelines include a table or chart of the weight ranges currently believed to be most healthful. (To find out how to get a copy of the *Dietary Guidelines for Americans*, see the RESOURCES section before the index of this book.)

Figure 1-1 shows the weight graph from the 1995 *Dietary Guidelines for Americans*. You'll notice that it's hard to tell precisely where the boundary between healthy weight and overweight falls. The Dietary Guidelines Advisory Committee blurred the boundaries on purpose. It wanted to stress that these categories do not have sharp edges. If you're near a border, you may prefer a clear, definitive answer about which side you fall on. But in reality, a pound more or less does not make the difference between being a healthy weight and being overweight.

Body Mass Index

Another guide to the healthiness of your weight is the body mass index, often called the BMI. To figure yours:

FIGURE 1-1

Are You Overweight?

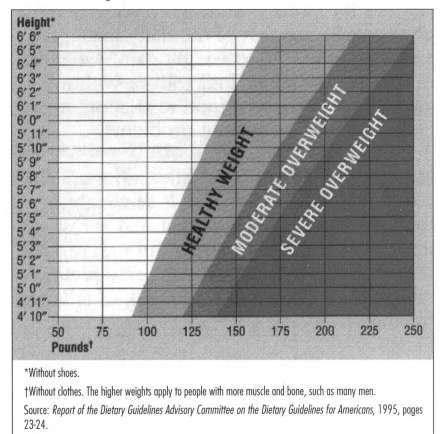

*Without shoes.

†Without clothes. The higher weights apply to people with more muscle and bone, such as many men.

Source: *Report of the Dietary Guidelines Advisory Committee on the Dietary Guidelines for Americans*, 1995, pages 23-24.

1. Multiply your weight in pounds by 705.

2. Divide your answer by your height in inches.

3. Take the answer and divide it by your height again.

Or, if you don't want to do the calculations yourself, just look at Table 1-1. This table also has heavy lines to show you where the boundaries between the various weight categories of Figure 1-1 fall. Remember, these

TABLE 1-1

Your Body Mass Index (BMI) and the Weight Guidelines of the *Dietary Guidelines for Americans*

Find the column with your height and the row with your weight. Where this column and row intersect is your BMI. For example, if you are 68 inches tall and weigh 170 pounds, your BMI is 25.9. The heavy lines mark the same divisions as in Figure 1-1, where BMIs of 20 to 25 are considered a "healthy weight," BMIs of 25 to 29 indicate "moderate overweight," and BMIs above 29 indicate "severe overweight."

WEIGHT (POUNDS)	58	59	60 (5 FEET)	61	62	63	64	65	66	67	HEIGHT (INCHES) 68	69	70	71	72 (6 FEET)	73	74	75	76	77	78	79	80
100	20.9	20.2	19.6	18.9	18.3	17.8	17.2	16.7	16.2	15.7	15.2	14.8	14.4	14.0	13.6	13.2	12.9	12.5	12.2	11.9	11.6	11.3	11.0
105	22.0	21.3	20.5	19.9	19.2	18.6	18.1	17.5	17.0	16.5	16.0	15.5	15.1	14.7	14.3	13.9	13.5	13.2	12.8	12.5	12.2	11.9	11.6
110	23.0	22.3	21.5	20.8	20.2	19.5	18.9	18.3	17.8	17.3	16.8	16.3	15.8	15.4	14.9	14.5	14.2	13.8	13.4	13.1	12.7	12.4	12.1
115	24.1	23.3	22.5	21.8	21.1	20.4	19.8	19.2	18.6	18.0	17.5	17.0	16.5	16.1	15.6	15.2	14.8	14.4	14.0	13.7	13.3	13.0	12.7
120	25.1	24.3	23.5	22.7	22.0	21.3	20.6	20.0	19.4	18.8	18.3	17.8	17.3	16.8	16.3	15.9	15.4	15.0	14.6	14.3	13.9	13.5	13.2
125	26.2	25.3	24.5	23.7	22.9	22.2	21.5	20.8	20.2	19.6	19.0	18.5	18.0	17.5	17.0	16.5	16.1	15.7	15.2	14.9	14.5	14.1	13.8
130	27.2	26.3	25.4	24.6	23.8	23.1	22.4	21.7	21.0	20.4	19.8	19.2	18.7	18.2	17.7	17.2	16.7	16.3	15.9	15.4	15.1	14.7	14.3
135	28.3	27.3	26.4	25.6	24.7	24.0	23.2	22.5	21.8	21.2	20.6	20.0	19.4	18.9	18.3	17.8	17.4	16.9	16.5	16.0	15.6	15.2	14.9
140	29.3	28.3	27.4	26.5	25.7	24.9	24.1	23.3	22.6	22.0	21.3	20.7	20.1	19.6	19.0	18.5	18.0	17.5	17.1	16.6	16.2	15.8	15.4
145	30.4	29.3	28.4	27.5	26.6	25.7	24.9	24.2	23.5	22.8	22.1	21.5	20.8	20.3	19.7	19.2	18.7	18.2	17.7	17.2	16.8	16.4	16.0
150	31.4	30.4	29.4	28.4	27.5	26.6	25.8	25.0	24.3	23.5	22.9	22.2	21.6	21.0	20.4	19.8	19.3	18.8	18.3	17.8	17.4	16.9	16.5
155	32.5	31.4	30.3	29.3	28.4	27.5	26.7	25.8	25.1	24.3	23.6	22.9	22.3	21.7	21.1	20.5	19.9	19.4	18.9	18.4	17.9	17.5	17.1
160	33.5	32.4	31.3	30.3	29.3	28.4	27.5	26.7	25.9	25.1	24.4	23.7	23.0	22.4	21.7	21.2	20.6	20.0	19.5	19.0	18.5	18.1	17.6
165	34.6	33.4	32.3	31.2	30.2	29.3	28.4	27.5	26.7	25.9	25.1	24.4	23.7	23.1	22.4	21.8	21.2	20.7	20.1	19.6	19.1	18.6	18.2
170	35.6	34.4	33.3	32.2	31.2	30.2	29.2	28.3	27.5	26.7	25.9	25.2	24.4	23.8	23.1	22.5	21.9	21.3	20.7	20.2	19.7	19.2	18.7
175	36.7	35.4	34.2	33.1	32.1	31.1	30.1	29.2	28.3	27.5	26.7	25.9	25.2	24.5	23.8	23.1	22.5	21.9	21.3	20.8	20.3	19.8	19.3
180	37.7	36.4	35.2	34.1	33.0	32.0	31.0	30.0	29.1	28.3	27.4	26.6	25.9	25.2	24.5	23.8	23.2	22.5	22.0	21.4	20.8	20.3	19.8

185	38.7	37.4	36.2	35.0	33.9	32.8	31.8	30.8	29.9	29.0	28.2	27.4	26.6	25.9	25.1	24.5	23.8	23.2	22.6	22.0	21.4	20.9	20.4
190	39.8	38.5	37.2	36.0	34.8	33.7	32.7	31.7	30.7	29.8	28.9	28.1	27.3	26.6	25.8	25.1	24.4	23.8	23.2	22.6	22.0	21.4	20.9
195	40.8	39.5	38.2	36.9	35.7	34.6	33.5	32.5	31.5	30.6	29.7	28.9	28.0	27.3	26.5	25.8	25.1	24.4	23.8	23.2	22.6	22.0	21.5
200	41.9	40.5	39.1	37.9	36.7	35.5	34.4	33.4	32.3	31.4	30.5	29.6	28.8	28.0	27.2	26.4	25.7	25.1	24.4	23.8	23.2	22.6	22.0
205	42.9	41.5	40.1	38.8	37.6	36.4	35.3	34.2	33.2	32.2	31.2	30.3	29.5	28.7	27.9	27.1	26.4	25.7	25.0	24.4	23.7	23.1	22.6
210	44.0	42.5	41.1	39.8	38.5	37.3	36.1	35.0	34.0	33.0	32.0	31.1	30.2	29.4	28.5	27.8	27.0	26.3	25.6	25.0	24.3	23.7	23.1
215	45.0	43.5	42.1	40.7	39.4	38.2	37.0	35.9	34.8	33.7	32.8	31.8	30.9	30.0	29.2	28.4	27.7	26.9	26.2	25.5	24.9	24.3	23.7
220	46.1	44.5	43.1	41.7	40.3	39.1	37.8	36.7	35.6	34.5	33.5	32.6	31.6	30.7	29.9	29.1	28.3	27.6	26.8	26.1	25.5	24.8	24.2
225	47.1	45.5	44.0	42.6	41.2	39.9	38.7	37.5	36.4	35.3	34.3	33.3	32.4	31.4	30.6	29.7	28.9	28.2	27.4	26.7	26.1	25.4	24.8
230	48.2	46.6	45.0	43.5	42.2	40.8	39.6	38.4	37.2	36.1	35.0	34.0	33.1	32.1	31.3	30.4	29.6	28.8	28.1	27.3	26.6	26.0	25.3
235	49.2	47.6	46.0	44.5	43.1	41.7	40.4	39.2	38.0	36.9	35.8	34.8	33.8	32.8	31.9	31.1	30.2	29.4	28.7	27.9	27.2	26.5	25.9
240	50.3	48.6	47.0	45.4	44.0	42.6	41.3	40.0	38.8	37.7	36.6	35.5	34.5	33.5	32.6	31.7	30.9	30.1	29.3	28.5	27.8	27.1	26.4
245	51.3	49.6	47.9	46.4	44.9	43.5	42.1	40.9	39.6	38.5	37.3	36.3	35.2	34.2	33.3	32.4	31.5	30.7	29.9	29.1	28.4	27.7	27.0
250	52.4	50.6	48.9	47.3	45.8	44.4	43.0	41.7	40.4	39.2	38.1	37.0	35.9	34.9	34.0	33.1	32.2	31.3	30.5	29.7	29.0	28.2	27.5
255	53.4	51.6	49.9	48.3	46.7	45.3	43.9	42.5	41.2	40.0	38.9	37.7	36.7	35.6	34.7	33.7	32.8	31.9	31.1	30.3	29.5	28.8	28.1
260	54.5	52.6	50.9	49.2	47.7	46.2	44.7	43.4	42.1	40.8	39.6	38.5	37.4	36.3	35.3	34.4	33.5	32.6	31.7	30.9	30.1	29.4	28.6
265	55.5	53.6	51.9	50.2	48.6	47.0	45.6	44.2	42.9	41.6	40.4	39.2	38.1	37.0	36.0	35.0	34.1	33.2	32.3	31.5	30.7	29.9	29.2
270	56.5	54.6	52.8	51.1	49.5	47.9	46.4	45.0	43.7	42.4	41.1	40.0	38.8	37.7	36.7	35.7	34.7	33.8	32.9	32.1	31.3	30.5	29.7
275	57.6	55.7	53.8	52.1	50.4	48.8	47.3	45.9	44.5	43.2	41.9	40.7	39.5	38.4	37.4	36.4	35.4	34.4	33.5	32.7	31.8	31.0	30.3
280	58.6	56.7	54.8	53.0	51.3	49.7	48.2	46.7	45.3	43.9	42.7	41.4	40.3	39.1	38.1	37.0	36.0	35.1	34.2	33.3	32.4	31.6	30.8
285	59.7	57.7	55.8	54.0	52.2	50.6	49.0	47.5	46.1	44.7	43.4	42.2	41.0	39.8	38.7	37.7	36.7	35.7	34.8	33.9	33.0	32.2	31.4
290	60.7	58.7	56.8	54.9	53.2	51.5	49.9	48.4	46.9	45.5	44.2	42.9	41.7	40.5	39.4	38.3	37.3	36.3	35.4	34.5	33.6	32.7	31.9
295	61.8	59.7	57.7	55.9	54.1	52.4	50.7	49.2	47.7	46.3	44.9	43.7	42.4	41.2	40.1	39.0	38.0	36.9	36.0	35.1	34.2	33.3	32.5
300	62.8	60.7	58.7	56.8	55.0	53.3	51.6	50.0	48.5	47.1	45.7	44.4	43.1	41.9	40.8	39.7	38.6	37.6	36.6	35.6	34.7	33.9	33.0
305	63.9	61.7	59.7	57.7	55.9	54.1	52.5	50.9	49.3	47.9	46.5	45.1	43.9	42.6	41.5	40.3	39.2	38.2	37.2	36.2	35.3	34.4	33.6
310	64.9	62.7	60.7	58.7	56.8	55.0	53.3	51.7	50.1	48.7	47.2	45.9	44.6	43.3	42.1	41.0	39.9	38.8	37.8	36.8	35.9	35.0	34.1
315	66.0	63.8	61.6	59.6	57.7	55.9	54.2	52.5	50.9	49.4	48.0	46.6	45.3	44.0	42.8	41.6	40.5	39.5	38.4	37.4	36.5	35.6	34.7
320	67.0	64.8	62.6	60.6	58.7	56.8	55.0	53.4	51.8	50.2	48.8	47.4	46.0	44.7	43.5	42.3	41.2	40.1	39.0	38.0	37.1	36.1	35.2

Continued

TABLE 1-1 *Continued*

Your Body Mass Index (BMI) and the Weight Guidelines of the *Dietary Guidelines for Americans*

Find the column with your height and the row with your weight. Where this column and row intersect is your BMI. For example, if you are 68 inches tall and weigh 170 pounds, your BMI is 25.9. The heavy lines mark the same divisions as in Figure 1-1, where BMIs of 20 to 25 are considered a "healthy weight," BMIs of 25 to 29 indicate "moderate overweight," and BMIs above 29 indicate "severe overweight."

										HEIGHT (INCHES)													
WEIGHT (POUNDS)	58	59	60 (5 FEET)	61	62	63	64	65	66	67	68	69	70	71	72 (6 FEET)	73	74	75	76	77	78	79	80
325	68.1	65.8	63.6	61.5	59.6	57.7	55.9	54.2	52.6	51.0	49.5	48.1	46.7	45.4	44.2	43.0	41.8	40.7	39.6	38.6	37.6	36.7	35.8
330	69.1	66.8	64.6	62.5	60.5	58.6	56.8	55.0	53.4	51.8	50.3	48.8	47.4	46.1	44.8	43.6	42.5	41.3	40.3	39.2	38.2	37.3	36.3
335	70.2	67.8	65.6	63.4	61.4	59.5	57.6	55.9	54.2	52.6	51.0	49.6	48.2	46.8	45.5	44.3	43.1	42.0	40.9	39.8	38.8	37.8	36.9
340	71.2	68.8	66.5	64.4	62.3	60.4	58.5	56.7	55.0	53.4	51.8	50.3	48.9	47.5	46.2	45.0	43.7	42.6	41.5	40.4	39.4	38.4	37.4
345	72.3	69.8	67.5	65.3	63.2	61.2	59.3	57.5	55.8	54.1	52.6	51.1	49.6	48.2	46.9	45.6	44.4	43.2	42.1	41.0	40.0	38.9	38.0
350	73.3	70.8	68.5	66.3	64.1	62.1	60.2	58.4	56.6	54.9	53.3	51.8	50.3	48.9	47.6	46.3	45.0	43.8	42.7	41.6	40.5	39.5	38.5
355	74.4	71.9	69.5	67.2	65.1	63.0	61.1	59.2	57.4	55.7	54.1	52.5	51.0	49.6	48.2	46.9	45.7	44.5	43.3	42.2	41.1	40.1	39.1
360	75.4	72.9	70.5	68.2	66.0	63.9	61.9	60.0	58.2	56.5	54.9	53.3	51.8	50.3	48.9	47.6	46.3	45.1	43.9	42.8	41.7	40.6	39.6
365	76.4	73.9	71.4	69.1	66.9	64.8	62.8	60.9	59.0	57.3	55.6	54.0	52.5	51.0	49.6	48.3	47.0	45.7	44.5	43.4	42.3	41.2	40.2
370	77.5	74.9	72.4	70.1	67.8	65.7	63.6	61.7	59.8	58.1	56.4	54.8	53.2	51.7	50.3	48.9	47.6	46.3	45.1	44.0	42.8	41.8	40.7
375	78.5	75.9	73.4	71.0	68.7	66.6	64.5	62.5	60.7	58.9	57.1	55.5	53.9	52.4	51.0	49.6	48.2	47.0	45.7	44.6	43.4	42.3	41.3
380	79.6	76.9	74.4	72.0	69.6	67.5	65.4	63.4	61.5	59.6	57.9	56.2	54.6	53.1	51.6	50.2	48.9	47.6	46.4	45.2	44.0	42.9	41.8
385	80.6	77.9	75.3	72.9	70.6	68.3	66.2	64.2	62.3	60.4	58.7	57.0	55.4	53.8	52.3	50.9	49.5	48.2	47.0	45.7	44.6	43.5	42.4
390	81.7	78.9	76.3	73.8	71.5	69.2	67.1	65.0	63.1	61.2	59.4	57.7	56.1	54.5	53.0	51.6	50.2	48.8	47.6	46.3	45.2	44.0	42.9
395	82.7	79.9	77.3	74.8	72.4	70.1	67.9	65.9	63.9	62.0	60.2	58.5	56.8	55.2	53.7	52.2	50.8	49.5	48.2	46.9	45.7	44.6	43.5
400	83.8	81.0	78.3	75.7	73.3	71.0	68.8	66.7	64.7	62.8	60.9	59.2	57.5	55.9	54.4	52.9	51.5	50.1	48.8	47.5	46.3	45.2	44.0

boundaries are not as precise as they look. They are still just guidelines, not hard-and-fast rules for how much any particular person should weigh.

Most experts agree that a BMI of 25 should be the dividing line between a healthy weight and overweight. But scientists don't agree about where the boundary between overweight and severe overweight should fall. The cut-off in the *Dietary Guidelines for Americans* falls at a BMI of 29. But many scientists think the cutoff should be lower, perhaps at 27 or 28. This dis-agreement explains why your classification by *Dietary Guidelines for Americans* chart may not jibe with other charts you've seen. In part, these disagreements occur because the riskiness of excess weight gradually increases as weight increases. Also, riskiness varies with each disease. That is, a weight that's risky for someone with diabetes may not be as risky for someone with a different disease. So whether you use the *Dietary Guidelines for Americans* or some other health organization's chart, you should take them as general guidelines only, not firm rules.

Keep in mind that these guidelines take into account only your height when suggesting a weight range. As Chapter 2 will show you, other traits matter as well. For example, a bodybuilder may be lean, yet because of large muscles may weigh more than the guidelines suggest. In contrast, an inactive person with a spare tire may be within the suggested weight range, yet have too much fat.

ATTITUDES ABOUT WEIGHT

You may have been surprised to see the wide range of weights that are healthy for people of a given height. Unfortunately, mixed-up ideas about weight are common. On the one hand, Americans revel in the richness of our soil and our crops. Most Americans eat better than even royalty of times past. On the other hand, in the midst of this plenty, we hold up the underfed look as the ideal of feminine beauty.

It's easy for social pressure to be thin to distort your ideas about what you should look like. As you choose a weight-loss goal, it's important to face your own biases against fat. Doing so will help you choose a healthy, doable goal for yourself.

Starvation Is Not Healthy or Normal

Television and magazines present an image of beauty that is grossly out of step with what average people look like. For example, almost all the women on television and in magazines are far thinner than average.

In real life, people come in a variety of shapes and sizes. Contrary to common belief, bodies cannot be molded to any shape desired. Some people are thin naturally. But most can achieve model thinness only by subsisting on near-starvation rations. This point is so important, we'll repeat it: Most people are not born to be thin. Even successful models have to work hard at it. Some exercise more than an hour a day and greatly restrict their food intake to look the way they do.

Ads and movies may make gauntness seem glamorous, but in real life it's not. People who are underfed don't do their best at work or at home. They're often weak and listless. Their hair may fall out. They may become irritable and lose interest in almost everything. Their life revolves around food.

To lose weight and keep it off, you must realize that there's no virtue in self-torture and no sin in joyful eating. Losing weight does require that you take in fewer calories than you have been—there's no getting around that. But it also requires that you keep up a program of healthful eating permanently. Sticking to a new lifestyle forever is possible only if you enjoy it.

Thinness Is Not the Secret to Happiness

Social pressures to be thin make some women hate their bodies. Even some top models believe their bodies aren't thin enough. Cindy Crawford reportedly thinks her feet and arms are too big, and Linda Evangelista supposedly wishes her rib cage were smaller.

Dieting has become so commonplace and routine that even some thin women purposely try to lose weight. Men are not immune to social ideals of thinness. Social pressure is increasing on them to look trim as well.

A lot of people stand to make a lot of money by convincing you that you would be happier if you looked different. It's no wonder that even some ads aimed at children stress improving their appearance.

Gluttony Is Not Healthy or Normal, Either

In the past, when people weren't blessed with the abundance of food we have now, people tended to feast on special occasions and eat sparingly the rest of the time. But today, every day has become a feast day.

A SHIFT IN VIEWPOINT

"When you are really obese, you feel like you're moving through mud all the time," says Gloria Friedrichson.* "I've been overweight since I was 8 years old. I've never had any luck in losing it and keeping it off."

It didn't help matters that magazine models were thin. "When I was young, I always wanted to be just like them, and I have been on severe diets in my life," Friedrichson says. "And of course, none of it ever helped because it's a diet—you go on it, you stay on it for a while, and then you go off."

Today, she attends a university weight-loss clinic and takes weight-loss drugs. She also exercises and follows the sensible meal plan the weight-loss program recommends: "We tried to maintain our daily caloric intake at about 1,500 calories and our fat gram intake at about 20% of our total calories. Otherwise, we were free to eat anything we wanted to—but if you eat processed foods and things that are heavily laden in fat, you can't eat much. You get hungry." So she eats a lot of vegetables and grains that make her feel more full. She has lost 49 pounds in a year and a half.

She found the secret to losing weight in her own head. "It took me many, many years to figure out that you just have to change your whole way of thinking about food," she says.

Many chapters of this book contain vignettes like this one. In them, you'll meet other people with diabetes who have long struggled with their weight. Although they are identified only by pseudonyms, their stories are otherwise completely true. Some have appeared previously in Diabetes Forecast.

Partly as a result of eating more food than they need, most people in the United States are overweight. The National Health and Nutrition Examination Survey conducted between 1991 and 1994 found that 59% of American men and 49% of American women have BMIs above 25.

One element of losing weight and keeping it off is rejecting the idea that it's normal and natural to eat until stuffed.

Ideas of Beauty Change

In recent years, scientists have begun exploring what makes people beautiful. They have found that some features are thought attractive by most people. For example, adults and babies alike seem to prefer symmetric faces (that is, faces in which the right side is close to being a mirror image of the left side).

But other aspects of beauty seem subject to the whims of fashion and personal taste. Which is more beautiful, straight hair or curly hair? Mustaches or clean-shaven upper lips? Tattooed skin or plain skin? Even within the 20th century, the answers have changed.

Which body size is most beautiful also changes. The Gibson Girl, with average measurements of 38-27-45, was considered slender and athletic-looking in the 1890s. And she **was** slim, compared with the plump women celebrated in Renaissance art by painters such as Peter Paul Rubens.

People come in a variety of sizes, and which size is thought most attractive changes. Being overweight when the fashion is to be very thin is no more a personality defect than is having straight hair when curly hair is the rage.

Overweight Is Not a Moral Failing

A lot of evidence suggests that some people just put on fat more easily than others. For example, people differ in how many calories they burn when they're not doing anything and in how many calories they burn after eating. People also differ in how much they're inclined to move around. Many of these differences seem to run in families. As a result, two people of the same height who eat the same diet may not weigh the same.

Some scientists believe that the "thrifty gene" theory, proposed in 1962 by James Neel, helps explain the origins of some diabetes and overweight. Neel pointed out that for most of human history, food was often scarce. People who burned calories frugally were at an advantage. They would store extra fat when food was plentiful and so be less likely to starve during famines. Today, the situation is reversed in Western countries. Most people have plenty of food available. People who conserve calories can put on a lot of weight if they eat more than their bodies need.

Having a natural inclination toward calorie frugality does not mean you're destined to be fat. People with thrifty genes still have choices about how much and what kind of food they eat and how active they are. They can choose to fight their tendency to gain weight. There's a good reason to try: Being overweight can cause all sorts of health problems. (You'll read about them in Chapter 4.) So it is worthwhile for people who gain weight easily to fight extra hard to keep pounds off.

THE MIDDLE COURSE

Extreme dieting is not healthful. Overeating is not healthful. These are not the only choices. Rather, the most healthful choice is the middle course.

The goal of this book is to help you find and follow that middle course: achieving a sensible, healthy weight and staying there. A sensible weight is not a weight at which you look like a model. It is not a weight where all your problems or guilty feelings over food miraculously fall away. It may not be the weight that's easiest for you to maintain.

So what is a healthy weight? A healthy weight means that you have achieved a balance. On the one hand, you are eating enough to function your best mentally and physically. On the other hand, you are at a weight at which you can keep your diabetes under control and avoid many health problems.

The linchpin of a healthy weight is a healthful diet. A healthful diet:

- Has the right balance of carbohydrates, fats, and proteins.

- Has enough nutrients to prevent deficiencies.

- Does not have too many calories.

Reading this book will not undo the damage of having lived many years with society's unrealistic expectations. But it's still important to be aware of social pressures and the messages of TV and magazine images. Setting these aside will help you choose a course that will make you healthier and happier.

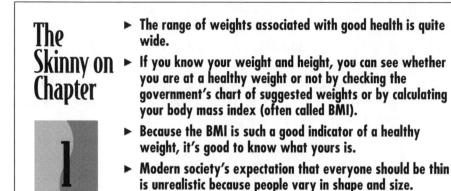

The
Skinny on
Chapter

1

▶ The range of weights associated with good health is quite wide.

▶ If you know your weight and height, you can see whether you are at a healthy weight or not by checking the government's chart of suggested weights or by calculating your body mass index (often called BMI).

▶ Because the BMI is such a good indicator of a healthy weight, it's good to know what yours is.

▶ Modern society's expectation that everyone should be thin is unrealistic because people vary in shape and size.

▶ Over time, ideas about which size is most attractive change.

▶ A sensible weight means that you are eating enough to function at your best mentally and physically, and you are at a weight at which you can keep your diabetes under control and avoid many health problems.

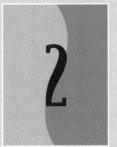

Be Yourself

Everyone's different. So target weights must be different, too.

Imagine the surprise and dismay around your living room if everyone opened a holiday present from you and found a size-large pink sweater. "Wrong color!" your brother says. "Wrong size!" your third-grade niece says. "Too hot!" your cousin from Florida says. "Too trendy!" your grandmother says. Perhaps only one recipient likes your gift—your dog, who has shredded his sweater and is now peacefully sleeping on a pile of pink yarn.

In real life, whether you're buying presents or serving guests at a dinner party, you don't give everyone the same thing. People come in different sexes, different ages, and different sizes. They have different tastes and different goals in life. You try to take these differences into account.

There are a lot of differences to take into account when you set a weight-loss goal, too. Table 1-1 shows the weights that researchers have found to be healthiest for the typical person. But just as one-size-fits-all pantyhose don't really fit everyone, neither do the standard weight tables. People differ in many ways, including their body shapes and how muscular they are. Weight tables can only be guides.

This chapter will help you think about what's unique about you and also help you choose a weight that's healthy for you.

ARE YOU AN APPLE OR A PEAR?

Scientists often divide people into "pears" and "apples." People who are pears tend to put on fat around their lower bodies (hips and thighs). People who are apples tend to put on fat around their upper bodies, waists, and abdomens.

It turns out that shape might be an important factor in how much you should weigh. Fat in some places may be more dangerous than fat in other places. So it could be more important for people with certain body shapes to lose weight.

Unfortunately, apples tend to have more health problems than pears:

- Apple-shaped people tend to be more resistant to the effects of insulin. Insulin resistance means that their bodies don't process glucose as well as they should. As a result, glucose levels can rise too high.

- Apples tend to have higher cholesterol levels.

- Apples are more likely to get heart and blood vessel disease.

- Apples are more likely to get high blood pressure.

You may notice that the conditions that are more common in apples are also more common in people with diabetes. It may be that type 2 diabetes and an apple shape are linked. People who collect fat around their middles do seem to be more likely to get type 2 diabetes.

It may be obvious when you look in the mirror whether you are an apple or a pear. On the other hand, you may think you most resemble a banana or a strawberry. Don't worry—there's a formula for figuring out whether you are more apple-like or pear-like. It's called the waist-to-hip ratio. To calculate yours:

1. Measure your waist. (Some bodies don't nip in at the waist. If you're unsure where your waist is, measure 1 inch above your navel.)

2. Measure your hips where they are biggest.

3. Divide your waist measurement by your hip measurement.

If you are a woman, you are an apple if your ratio is bigger than 0.8, and you are a pear if your ratio is less than 0.8.

If you are a man, you are an apple if your ratio is bigger than 1.0, and you are a pear if your ratio is less than 1.0.

PLEASURES AND PAINS OF OVEREATING

"There's security in being heavy," says Diane Prosper. "I can blame everything that I don't like about my life on my weight." Food plays many important roles in her life. "I believe that I eat for every reason other than physical hunger. I eat for comfort. I eat for happy. I eat for sad. I eat for lonely," she says. "The more sugar I have, the more comfortable I feel."

Despite these pleasures, Prosper's weight has caused her great sadness. Getting on the school bus as a child meant enduring taunts and jeers. "When I was in seventh grade, some five girls in the class decided that it would be their personal mission to make my seventh grade year miserable," she says. "They pretty well succeeded," playing such tricks as tossing her underwear in the shower after physical education class.

Adulthood had its own pains. "I have yet to ever go on a date or be approached by a male. Ever. And I'm going to be 40 next month," she says. She never flew in a plane until she was 39 for fear she couldn't squeeze into the seat. And she always worries about fitting into seats in meetings, in auditoriums, at movie theaters, and on the bus.

She is now trying hard to resist the lure of food so that she can lose weight and be healthy. "I recently was blessed to be able to adopt two children," she says. "And I want to live to see them grow up and graduate high school and college and get married and all of those wonderful things that I'm blessed enough to be able to do as a parent."

Genetics and getting older can influence your body shape, but so can your behavior and lifestyle. For example, smokers and inactive people are more likely to be apples.

HOW OLD ARE YOU?

After about age 35, many people start to put on extra body fat. This weight gain occurs even in people who exercise a lot. Worse yet, the older you are, the more likely it is that extra fat ends up on your abdomen. For these reasons, middle-aged people may want to try to get down to a lower weight than younger people.

Scientists are uncertain what a healthy weight for older people is. One reason is that once people get into their 60s, the weight gain that started about age 35 usually stops. After that, people tend to lose weight without making any effort to do so. This weight loss occurs partly because they are losing muscle and bone. Sickness can also wear people down and make them lose weight.

These factors hint that extra weight may not be quite as harmful to older people as to younger people. Even so, some doctors believe older people should strive for the same weight goals as younger people. If you are over 65 and think you may be overweight, you should discuss your options in detail with your doctor.

ARE YOU A MAN OR A WOMAN?

Men's and women's bodies tend to store fat differently and to need different amounts of fat.

Women tend to put on fat on their hips and buttocks. Men tend to put on fat on their upper body and abdomen. So women tend to be pears, and men, apples.

Sometimes people view fat as bad or evil. But in fact, having some fat is necessary for good health. The amount of fat needed varies greatly between men and women. A man can be healthy if fat makes up at least 3% of his weight (although 10% is a better lower limit). A woman needs fat to make up at least 12%, and possibly more, of her weight to be healthy. And more fat than that is probably needed for a woman to be able to get pregnant. At the upper end, women should not be more than 30%

fat, and men should not be more than 25% fat. But both sexes should try to achieve a weight and body mass index (BMI) in the normal range.

Pregnancy

Women with diabetes who are pregnant should not try to lose weight. On the contrary, the American Diabetes Association recommends that all women with diabetes gain weight during pregnancy.

Your doctor can best advise you how much weight to gain. Your change in weight will tell you whether you should increase or decrease your calories to reach your weight-gain goal.

If you did not develop diabetes until you were pregnant, how much weight you should gain is a more complex question. Getting diabetes when you are pregnant is called gestational diabetes. (You can read more about gestational diabetes in Chapter 17.) To have a healthy infant, you will need to bring your glucose level down. One way to lower blood glucose is to eat fewer calories. As a result, some doctors suggest that obese pregnant women with gestational diabetes cut calories so that they gain only a few pounds. Other doctors believe that women with gestational diabetes should gain about the same amount of weight as women who had diabetes before becoming pregnant. Again, your doctor can help you decide how much weight gain is best for you.

If you had diabetes while you were pregnant and it went away after your baby was born, you're not out of the woods. Having had gestational diabetes raises your risk of getting type 2 diabetes later in life: 30 to 40% of women who've had gestational diabetes get type 2 diabetes within a decade or two. Whether you do later get type 2 diabetes depends in part on your weight. Overweight women are more than twice as likely as normal-weight women to get type 2 diabetes.

Some women have trouble losing all their excess weight after their babies are born. In fact, for some women, a battle with extra pounds first starts during pregnancy. (See the box "Spotlight on Research: Pregnancy Pounds.")

Menopause

After menopause, female hormone levels drop. Women then deposit fat more as men do, on their abdomens and upper bodies. They also tend to put on weight at a faster rate than before.

SPOTLIGHT ON RESEARCH
Pregnancy Pounds

The Stockholm Pregnancy and Weight Development Study (reported in *Obesity Research* in 1995) looked at the tendency for some women's weight problems to start during pregnancy. Researchers weighed 1,423 women 1 year after they gave birth. The researchers then compared these weights with what the women had weighed before getting pregnant. The women averaged a net gain of only about 1 pound. But that average hides a lot of differences among the women. A third of the women weighed less than before getting pregnant. Another 14% or so had gained at least 11 pounds. In fact, some women lost as much as 26 pounds, and others gained as much as 57 pounds.

The Swedish researchers found the women who had the highest weight gains 1 year after pregnancy shared certain features. They were more likely than the other women to have gained a lot of weight while pregnant. They also were less likely to have breastfed their babies and more likely to have irregular eating habits, to skip breakfasts and lunches, and to be sedentary.

This study shows that:

- Although women should gain weight during pregnancy, they should try to stick to the suggested weight gain. Extra pounds could end up sticking around a long time.

- New babies change their mothers' lifestyles, and these changes can lead to weight gain. It's a good idea for new mothers to make an effort to eat regular, healthful meals and get some exercise, even though finding the time and energy to do so can be very hard.

These changes mean that it's harder for older women to get to or stay at a healthy weight. Yet, because of the greater risk of heart disease, it's even more important for older women to be at a healthy weight. Heart attack is the biggest killer of American women, killing about twice as many each year as all forms of cancer combined. Women with diabetes have a much higher risk of heart disease than other women. Taking hormones after menopause can improve a woman's risk factors for heart disease, but hormones may help diabetic women less.

For these reasons, it's extra important for women past menopause who want to lose weight to talk to their doctor and a dietitian.

ARE YOU MUSCULAR OR FLABBY?

Muscle weighs more than fat. This weight difference means that two people may be the same height and weight, yet only one person may be too fat. A scientist would say that both are overweight, but only one is obese. But not everyone's language is this precise. Often, "overweight" and "obese" are used as if they mean the same thing.

Arnold Schwarzenegger is a good example of the difference between overweight and obese. At the peak of his weight-lifting career, Schwarzenegger was 6 feet 2 inches tall and weighed 235 pounds. According to the chart of suggested weights in the *Dietary Guidelines for Americans* (Figure 1-1), a person this tall should weigh between 148 and 194 pounds. Schwarzenegger was clearly overweight. He was 41 pounds above the maximum healthy weight for his height. But he was not obese because he did not have too much body fat.

The opposite can sometimes happen, too. A small-boned, naturally thin person who puts on a lot of fat may be obese despite falling within the suggested weight range.

As a result, flabby and small-boned people usually need to aim for a lower weight than muscular and big-boned people.

HAVE YOU GAINED WEIGHT OVER TIME?

According to the *Dietary Guidelines for Americans,* if you fall within the weight ranges recommended for your height (Figure 1-1, Table 1-1), you don't need to lose weight. But the guidelines make an exception for people who have gained more than 10 pounds since reaching their adult height. Other experts stress that people who gain even 5 to 10 pounds in adulthood should take immediate steps to lose it.

Of course, it matters whether those pounds are fat or muscle. If you've added muscle because you are a miner or lumberjack or have some other physically demanding job, that's one thing. But if your new pounds fall mostly in the padding category, you should talk to your doctor about possibly losing weight even if your weight falls in the healthful range. If you have type 2 diabetes, then losing these few pounds could make a big difference in your glucose control.

DO YOU HAVE TYPE 1 DIABETES?

Many people with type 1 diabetes are now working on tight control. Tight control means that a person is aiming for a blood glucose level in the normal range and is doing a variety of things to achieve it. These include measuring blood glucose several times a day and using an insulin pump or taking several insulin injections a day.

Weight gain is a frequent side effect of tight control. People who go on tight control gain an average of about 10 pounds. In the past, many people with type 1 diabetes did not need to worry about their weight. But with tight control, more and more people with type 1 may face a weight gain.

Little research has yet been done on the relationship between weight and mortality in people with type 1 diabetes. Scientists need to find out whether gaining a little weight with tight control is harmful. Probably, though, people with type 1 whose weight is above the healthy range should consider losing weight, just like anyone else. And of course, improving glucose control to cut the chances of complications is vital.

IS YOUR WEIGHT CAUSING YOU PROBLEMS NOW?

Being overweight can cause many health problems. (We'll go into the gruesome details in Chapter 4.) But not everyone suffers equally from their weight. Some overweight people manage to avoid many weight-related health problems.

Because you have diabetes, you're not in that group. Type 2 diabetes is considered a weight-related problem because overweight people are far more likely to get this form of diabetes. And no matter what kind of diabetes you have, your glucose levels are affected by how much you weigh, what you eat, and how active you are. Adopting a healthful lifestyle will most likely help you control your glucose better.

But how else is your weight affecting you? Your answer affects how much weight you may want to try to lose. For example, if you have arthritis in your knees or hips, you may want to lose as much weight as you can. The less you weigh, the less burden your tender joints will have to bear. On the other hand, if you have no weight-related condition other than diabetes, you may prefer to lose only as much weight as you need to bring your diabetes under good control.

People who have weight-related health problems, including diabetes, should talk to their doctors before starting a weight-loss program. It's extra important for them to choose a safe food plan and exercise program.

WILL YOUR WEIGHT CAUSE PROBLEMS IN THE FUTURE?

Even if you are not suffering now from your weight, your family history could make problems more likely in the future. What diseases have your closest relatives (parents, grandparents, brothers, sisters, and children) had? Do conditions such as heart attack, stroke, blood vessel problems, high cholesterol, or high blood pressure run in your family? Overweight plays a role in these conditions. Preventing further weight gain can help to slow their development. Losing weight can be even more important in helping you avoid or delay getting these diseases yourself.

The Skinny on Chapter

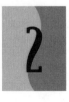

▶ The healthy-weight charts are meant for the typical person. The best weight for you may be at one end or another of the range—or even out of the range altogether.

▶ Fat on the hips and thighs may be less dangerous than fat on the waist and abdomen.

▶ An apple shape (with fat on waist and abdomen) is associated with higher cholesterol levels, insulin resistance, high blood pressure, and heart and blood vessel disease.

▶ Men, smokers, older people, sedentary people, and overweight people are more likely to have the less-healthy apple shape.

Continued

The Skinny on Chapter 2
Continued

► Pregnant women with diabetes should not try to lose weight. But they should gain only as much as their doctor advises.

► People typically start putting on weight in middle age, but then may start losing it in their 60s.

► People who have weight-related health problems, including diabetes, should talk to their doctors before starting a weight-loss program.

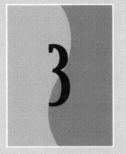

Select Your Goal

It's best to set your sights on a "reasonable" weight—one that improves your health and is within reach.

Wouldn't it be great if, like Goldilocks, we always knew exactly what was right for us? Goldilocks quickly rated all the bowls of porridge— "Too hot! Too cold! Just right!"—and then gobbled down the one that met her standards. She didn't hesitate in the bears' bedroom, either. One bed got a "Too hard!" One got a "Too soft!" And she pronounced the final bed "Just right!" before falling asleep in it.

If Goldilocks were choosing a weight-loss goal, you can bet she wouldn't aim too high or too low. She'd know which goal was "Just right!" But for most people who are trying to lose weight, it's not so easy. It's not always obvious whether a weight-loss goal is too ambitious or too humble. Yet the stakes are high. Your health and happiness are at risk if you set your sights too high or too low.

Chapters 1 and 2 talked about what a healthy weight is and how personal factors can influence your weight. Now it's time to choose a weight goal for yourself. This chapter will focus on setting a goal that combines three features:

- It will be possible for you to get down to that weight.

- Once you get down to that weight, your health will improve.

- It will be possible for you to stay at that weight.

DIABETES AND YOUR GOAL

An important thing to keep in mind when setting your goal is that your diabetes probably will improve if you just **try** to lose weight.

Notice that small but vital word "try." One surprising result of many studies has been that exercising and cutting the number of calories you eat can improve glucose levels—even if you lose little weight!

If you've ever tried to lose weight before, you may have noticed a pattern in your progress. You lose weight at first, then weight loss tapers off. Finally, you gain back all or most of what you lost. There are biological reasons for this pattern. Later chapters will talk about ways to avoid these problems.

In the meantime, keep in mind that the steps in this book are worth following for the rest of your life even if you don't take off much weight. They will help you control your glucose better. They will likely cut your risk of getting diseases linked to overweight. And, because most Americans gain weight as they get older, preventing weight gain is a great feat. It means you've done a lot to keep your glucose levels and disease risk factors from getting worse.

WHAT EXPERTS SUGGEST

The Ten-Percent Solution

Most scientists who study the effects of body weight think that losing as little as 10% to 15% of your weight can be enough to improve your health. This translates to 15 to 23 pounds for a person who weighs 150 pounds or 20 to 30 pounds for a 200-pound person. A 10% weight loss is often enough to improve high blood pressure and levels of cholesterol and other blood fats. A 10% weight loss may also bring blood glucose levels down, sometimes to normal.

A DOSE OF REALITY

Diane Prosper's weight goal has changed over the years. "It used to be what the insurance charts say when I was younger and naïve. A person of my height and bone structure should weigh about 154," she says. But she became more realistic as she got older. "I decided that my goal is to be able to go into a store like JCPenney or Braun['s] or any of those other women's stores and be able to buy a size 18 right off the rack. When I can do that, I will be one happy camper!"

For Better Health

You may want a more ambitious goal than losing 10% of your weight. You may want to get rid of all your excess weight and all the excess health risks your weight poses for you.

You already learned in Chapter 1 that overweight is often defined as a body mass index (BMI) above 25. This number was chosen because most health risks rise as BMI climbs above 25.

Because BMIs below 25 seem to be the healthiest, some experts suggest that overweight people try to lose enough weight to get down to a BMI of 25 or lower.

TORTOISES AND HARES

Whatever weight-loss goal you choose, slow and steady is the way to go.

It's common for people to try to lose a lot of weight in a brief time to be thin for a specific event—the start of bikini season or their wedding or high school reunion, for example. So they may try crash diets or other short-term fixes.

But too-rapid weight loss has dangers. Cutting back severely on how much you eat does more than make you feel hungry and irritable all the time. You may not get as much protein or vitamins as your body needs. You might get gallstones. Some people lose their hair or feel tired. There's even some evidence that food deprivation may trigger eating disorders in some people.

Even if you ignore the health danger of drastic diets, they still have a big drawback: The weight loss doesn't last. Temporary dieting is only a temporary fix. Striving for a healthy weight needs to be a lifetime habit, not a brief phase. If you adopt healthful habits for 3 months, then go back to your old ways of eating once you've lost 10 pounds, you'll almost certainly gain back the weight.

Lifelong healthful habits will let you lose weight now and will prevent or slow weight regain later. You might lose weight more slowly than if you did something drastic. But 5 years from now, 10 years from now, or 20 years from now, you'll weigh less if you live a healthful lifestyle than if you follow a temporary lose-weight-quick plan.

A good maximum weight loss for most people is 1 1/2 to 2 pounds a week. If this rate sounds slow, do a little math and see how those pounds add up over time. For example, if you lose 1 pound a week for 6 months, that adds up to 26 pounds.

Remember, it may have taken you decades to put on your excess pounds. If it takes you a few years to lose them, they're still coming off a lot faster than they went on.

WHY CHOOSE A REASONABLE WEIGHT-LOSS GOAL?

If you've been dreaming of buying a new wardrobe of size-6 clothes, the idea of trying for a sensible weight, not an ideal weight, may be disappointing. It may even seem a cop-out.

It's not. Although you can shrink fat cells, neither losing weight nor exercising can get rid of them entirely. The truth is, for most people who have a BMI of 40, trying to get to a BMI of 20 would be an impossible mission. But most people with a BMI of 40 are capable of losing enough weight to improve their health and to let them move with greater ease and comfort.

Setting a practical, doable weight-loss goal—say, to lose 10% of your current weight—has four advantages.

- Your chance of success is high. Although people vary in how much weight they lose on a weight-loss program, 10% is an average loss.

- You're more likely to be able to keep the weight off. If you set a goal of losing 50% of your weight, you may be able to do it. But keeping it off may prove too hard.

- You'll be healthier. Many studies show that weight loss of only 10% is enough to help blood pressure, cholesterol levels, and glucose levels. In fact, some people show improvement after losing only 5 or 10 pounds.

- You'll feel successful. Setting an unrealistic goal just means you'll spend a lot of time berating yourself for not achieving something that may have been impossible from the start.

Keep in mind that you can always set new goals for yourself. In fact, some experts believe that even if you want to lose a lot of weight, it's still best to set a modest goal for your first round, perhaps as little as 10 to 15 pounds. Once you've achieved that goal, you can then decide whether you want to set a new goal.

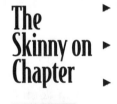

The
Skinny on
Chapter

3

▶ Even modest weight loss can reduce your risk of many diseases.

▶ If you have type 2 diabetes, losing weight is likely to bring your glucose levels down.

▶ Losing 10% of weight is a good goal for most overweight people. This amount is often enough to reduce your risk of weight-related diseases.

▶ A more ambitious goal is to get down to a BMI of 25. This amount of weight loss will put your weight in the normal range and may get rid of most of the extra health risks your weight poses.

▶ Some experts suggest a stepped weight-loss approach, in which you alternate losing a modest amount with periods in which you make sure you can maintain that weight.

▶ There's usually no need to be in a hurry to drop weight.

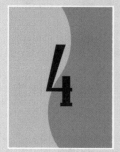
Defeating Diabetes and Other Weight-Related Problems

A healthful lifestyle can prevent many ailments. It may also help afflictions you already have.

Warning: This chapter is not upbeat. It details all the scary stuff that can happen when you weigh too much.

The goal of this chapter is not to frighten you, but to help you. Losing weight takes effort and commitment. This chapter will show you why all that work is worth it and help you see how even small changes in your life can make big changes in how happy and healthy you are.

A CHAIN REACTION

Knock over the first domino in a row of dominoes, and what happens? That domino knocks over a second, which knocks over a third, which knocks over a fourth, and so on until no dominoes are left standing.

Being overweight is like knocking over that first domino. It can start a chain reaction. For example, excess weight can raise the amount of some kinds of fat in your blood, which in turn can clog your arteries, which in turn can lead to heart attacks and strokes.

There's a good side to this chain reaction. Just as you can stop the dominoes from falling by removing one or two, making a few changes in your lifestyle can interrupt the cascade of health problems started by overweight. If you can reduce your weight by eating more healthfully and being more active, you can reduce your risk of heart disease, stroke, cancer, arthritis, and many other conditions. You will improve your diabetes. You may live longer. And you certainly will live more comfortably and enjoyably.

A HEALTHY HEART

Your heart is an incredibly strong organ. Although it weighs less than a pound, it pumps 2,500 gallons of blood every day. It beats 37 million times a year, never taking a rest.

Despite being encased inside your ribs, your heart is still vulnerable. Your choices in life can affect its health and future. In particular, aerobic exercise can make your heart strong, while being a couch potato allows it to weaken. Mental stress can be wearing on the heart. And the food you eat affects your blood and blood vessels and so affects your heart.

There is a whole slew of heart and blood vessel diseases.

Heart Attack. A heart attack happens when blood flow to the heart is cut off, usually because an artery is clogged. Heart muscle, starved for blood, then starts to die. The medical term for heart attack is "myocardial infarction."

Angina. Angina is a warning sign that a person is at risk of a heart attack. It consists of chest pain, usually during exercise.

Stroke. A stroke happens when blood flow to a part of the brain is cut off, often because an artery is clogged. Brain cells, starved for blood, then start to die.

Atherosclerosis. Atherosclerosis means that the arteries are clogged with cholesterol and other fats. Atherosclerosis can lead to heart attack and stroke.

Being overweight increases your risk of heart and blood vessel diseases in two ways:

- Being overweight increases your risk of high blood pressure and high levels of "bad" blood fats.

- Being overweight can make it harder to exercise. If your weight keeps you from exercising, your heart may not be as strong as it could be.

High Blood Pressure

High blood pressure (hypertension) is a condition that means exactly what its name implies: Blood is pressing harder against the walls of the arteries than it should. Just as a raging river cuts a channel through rock faster than a meandering stream does, blood flowing at high pressure is harder on your blood vessels than blood flowing at normal pressure. Over time, the extra wear and tear can damage blood vessels and some organs. As a result, too-high blood pressure puts you at risk of stroke, heart attack, eye disease, and kidney failure.

High blood pressure can result from many things. For example, blood pressure tends to rise as people get older. People who drink a lot of alcohol or who are inactive tend to have higher blood pressures.

The major cause of high blood pressure is overweight. Excess weight causes 30% to 50% of cases of high blood pressure. Not everyone who is overweight has high blood pressure. But people who are overweight are two to five times as likely as other people to have high blood pressure. Losing as little as 7 to 11 pounds can bring blood pressure down.

Blood Fats

Your blood contains fats that serve a variety of purposes. A high level of one of these fats is good for you. This fat is high-density lipoprotein (HDL) cholesterol ("good" cholesterol). People with high levels of HDL cholesterol have a lower risk of heart and vessel disease than do people with lower levels. People who are overweight tend to have less of this good fat.

Other fats seem unhealthy. At least, people with high levels are more likely to get heart and blood vessel disease. These fats include:

- Triglycerides

- Low-density lipoprotein (LDL) cholesterol ("bad" cholesterol)

- Total cholesterol (which includes both good HDL and less-healthful forms of cholesterol such as LDL)

People who are overweight tend to have more of the bad fats.

When Heart Disease Risk Factors Occur Together

People who have one risk factor for heart disease tend to have others. These risk factors are:

- Obesity (especially in the upper body)

- Insulin resistance (when the body does not respond to insulin as it should)

- Diabetes

- High blood pressure

- Atherosclerosis

- High triglyceride levels

- Low HDL cholesterol levels

- High LDL cholesterol levels

There is one silver lining to the clustering of heart disease risk factors. When you lose weight to improve one of these risk factors, you often improve them all.

GALLSTONES

Gallstones are more common in people who are obese. While a person is losing weight, the risk of getting gallstones actually goes up. Researchers believe slow weight loss may cause fewer gallstone problems than rapid weight loss. In any case, the rise in risk during weight loss is not permanent. After a person has reached a new, stable lower weight, gallstones become less likely. So losing weight will probably cut your risk of gallbladder problems over the long term.

BREATHING PROBLEMS

You may have heard an overweight person described as being smothered in fat. This is not just a figure of speech. Extra fat can indeed press on the lungs and make it hard to pull in enough air.

A sleeping problem called sleep apnea occurs more often in overweight people. People with sleep apnea have brief periods in which they stop breathing. They may wake up gasping and choking, sometimes several times a night. Losing weight takes pressure off the breathing apparatus and lets people sleep peacefully again.

CANCER

People who are overweight are more likely than other people to get certain kinds of cancers. Scientists don't really know what causes these extra cancers. It might be having extra body fat. It might be the changes in hormone levels that are common in overweight people. Or a high-calorie or high-fat diet might be the culprit: Like any other tissue in the body, cancer requires a lot of energy to grow.

Cancers probably have a variety of causes, and not every cancer is related to weight. Colon cancer, breast cancer, and endometrial cancer (cancer of the lining of the uterus) are the cancers most often associated with being overweight. (Studies also link some of these cancers with the amount of fat eaten.) Some other cancers may also be more common in obese people.

Some studies suggest that reducing calorie intake can reduce the chances of getting cancers.

ARTHRITIS

Extra pounds weigh heavily on the joints. Joints that are bearing more weight than they are designed to support can hurt—and may even wear down. Overweight people can suffer from several different joint problems.

People who are obese are more likely to have back pain than other people are.

People who are overweight are also more likely to have osteoarthritis. This form of arthritis occurs when cartilage breaks down and bone grinds against bone in the joint.

As you might expect, the greater the excess weight, the greater the pain in the joints. But when people lose weight, their joints should hurt less, and they can do more without pain. For some people, losing weight gets rid of all their joint pain. Losing weight can often prevent osteoarthritis

IN THE DEPTHS OF DESPAIR

Hazel Gilberti had always been a successful dieter—successful on grapefruit diets, liquid diets, doctor-supervised diets. With one weight-reduction program, she lost 114 pounds in 9 months. Then she gained 135 over the next 6 months.

"That's what I did constantly," she says. "I'd join programs with the very best intentions. In the first 2 weeks, I'd lose 11 pounds. The third week I'd gain 2. The fourth week, gain 3. All of a sudden, I'd be back to my original weight and then start gaining on the program."

At age 38, at a weight of 244, Gilberti was diagnosed with type 2 diabetes. She controlled it with diet and exercise at first.

"But, of course, I didn't adhere to it," she says. "I ended up on insulin within a year and, without a doctor's permission, was altering the dose as I kept eating. If I ate a dozen candy bars, I just took a little more insulin."

Gilberti eventually got up to 70 units of insulin a day and a weight of 287. "I had reached the saturation point. I just started eating, and I didn't give a darn, because for every weight loss that I was successful with, I was very unsuccessful keeping it off. If I lost a pound, I gained a pound and a quarter back. And the older I got, the more I gained. I couldn't combat it. I said, 'OK, I'm defeated.'"

The ending to Gilberti's story? You'll find out in Chapter 16.

if you do not already have it. One study found that losing as little as 11 pounds halved the risk of getting osteoarthritis of the knee later.

Gout is another form of arthritis that is more common in people who are overweight. Gout is not caused by the burden of extra weight on the bones. Instead, people who weigh more tend to have higher levels of uric acid. When levels of uric acid get high enough, crystals form. These crystals lodge in tissues around the joints. The big toe is one of the most frequently attacked joints.

When people lose weight, their uric acid levels may rise for a short time. Still, losing weight is part of the treatment for gout. Over time, uric acid levels may drop to normal.

DIABETES

Obesity and type 2 diabetes are tightly linked. The more overweight someone is, the higher his or her risk of getting diabetes is. Also, the longer a person has been overweight, the greater the risk. Obesity may sometimes lead to diabetes because of its effects on insulin resistance. Insulin is a hormone produced by the pancreas. Insulin's job is to help cells take glucose from the blood. Cells then use glucose for energy.

Sometimes, when people have too much fat, cells just don't respond well to insulin (insulin resistance). That is, cells don't take up glucose as quickly as they should. So glucose levels rise even though there may be lots of insulin in the blood. When glucose levels get high enough, the person is diagnosed with type 2 diabetes.

Because you already have diabetes, you may think that it's too late to worry about the link between overweight and diabetes. But in fact, it's not too late at all.

First, if you have type 2 diabetes, your children have a higher risk of diabetes just because they're related to you. The changes you make in your family's diet and activities to help you get to a healthier weight can help the rest of your family avoid diabetes.

Second, your weight can make a big difference in your diabetes control. Losing weight won't cure type 2 diabetes. But it will bring glucose levels down. Weight loss of 10 to 20 pounds can be enough to improve diabetes control. The closer to normal that people with diabetes keep their glucose levels, the fewer complications they tend to have.

The Diabetes Control and Complications Trial showed that good glucose control can greatly improve health. This study followed 1,441 people with type 1 diabetes for an average of 6 1/2 years. Half the people received the standard treatment for type 1 diabetes. This consisted of taking one or two shots of insulin each day, monitoring blood glucose every day, and learning about proper diet and exercise. The other half of the people were put on intensive treatment. They took three or more insulin doses each day and adjusted their insulin doses according to their glucose level, how active they expected to be, and what they expected to eat. These people also measured their glucose level at least four times a day. As a result of these treatment differences, people on intensive treatment kept their glucose levels much closer to normal.

SPOTLIGHT ON RESEARCH
Good Habits May Prevent Diabetes

A study of men in Malmö, Sweden, actively tried to prevent type 2 diabetes. The study appeared in *Diabetologia* in 1991. For 6 years, researchers followed 41 men whose type 2 diabetes had just been discovered by a blood test. These men did not yet have symptoms. The researchers also followed 181 men who had impaired glucose tolerance. (Impaired glucose tolerance means glucose levels are higher than normal, but not high enough to be called diabetes.) All of these men were invited to join a treatment program. Most accepted. They received advice about losing weight and began exercise programs.

In addition, the researchers chose other men as control subjects to receive no treatment. Of these men, 79 had impaired glucose tolerance and 114 had normal glucose levels.

At the end of the 6 years, the men in the treatment groups had lost and kept off a few pounds. In contrast, the average weight among the other men went up.

Of the men who had impaired glucose tolerance at the start and were in the treatment program, only 10% had progressed to diabetes. Most of the rest had improved their glucose levels. In contrast, glucose levels had gotten worse in two-thirds of the control subjects with impaired glucose tolerance. And 29% had progressed to diabetes.

The treatment program was also helpful to the men who already had diabetes at the start. More than half now had their diabetes so well under control that their glucose levels had become normal.

This study suggests that losing weight and becoming better fit can delay or prevent diabetes in men with impaired glucose tolerance. These actions may also freeze new diabetes in place so that it does not progress. Best of all, the treatment program appeared not to be harmful. In fact, the death rate was higher in the groups who did not receive treatment.

The effects of tight glucose control were large. It greatly reduced the risk of getting diabetic eye disease, diabetic nerve disease, and diabetic kidney disease. In people who already had a complication, tight control slowed its progress.

As a result of this trial, tight control became the preferred treatment goal for many adults with type 1 diabetes. Even though no people with type 2 diabetes were in the Diabetes Control and Complications Trial, doctors believe that keeping glucose levels as close to normal as possible will cut those people's risk of complications, too. Many people with type 2 diabetes can achieve good control without taking insulin. In fact, good eating and exercise habits are so crucial for people with type 2 diabetes that they are considered the first therapies to try. Doctors only add diabetes pills or insulin shots if the meal plan and exercise program do not do a good enough job on their own.

LIFE SPAN

Given all the health problems that being overweight can cause, it probably won't come as a surprise that people who are overweight tend to die younger than other people.

A study of some people who live in Framingham, Massachusetts, a small town near Boston, shows clearly how weight affects how long you live. The Framingham Study has been running since 1948. More than 5,000 men and women above the age of 30 have taken part. One goal of the study has been to follow the development of heart and blood vessel diseases in people who had none of these diseases to start with.

In a report of the Framingham results published in the *Journal of the American Medical Association* in 1988, researchers looked at older men and women. The report focused on 1,723 nonsmokers who lived to be at least age 65. Men and women were each divided into four groups based on their body mass index (BMI). The healthiest groups were men with BMIs between 23 and 25 and women with BMIs between 24 and 26. Compared with these people, the heaviest men (BMI greater than 28.5) were 70% more likely to die, and the heaviest women (BMI greater than 28.7) were 200% as likely (that is, twice as likely) to die. Men and women with BMIs between the healthy group and the heaviest group also had a higher risk of dying. In this study, the thinnest people had a higher death rate than the normal-weight people, possibly because the thin group contained people who were already sick. Like the many other reports on the Framingham Study, this one shows that being heavy can shorten your life span.

THE GOOD EFFECTS OF WEIGHT LOSS

The evidence is overwhelming that extra fat cheats you of a healthy life now and can rob years from your life later. Just showing that excess weight is often unhealthy does not necessarily mean that losing weight can improve the situation. But in fact, losing weight usually does improve health. Indeed, many studies suggest that even modest weight loss can make you healthier.

For example, a 1994 study in the *International Journal of Obesity and Related Metabolic Disorders* looked at the effects of modest weight loss on heart disease risk factors in men and women. The subjects were 101 men and 101 women from Pittsburgh and Minneapolis–St. Paul. All were healthy nonsmokers between 25 and 45 years old. They had no risk factors for heart disease, but were 30 to 70 pounds overweight. Some were given a manual on weight loss. The others went through a weight-control program that included weekly meetings, weigh-ins, calorie cutting, and exercise.

After 18 months, the subjects who received only a weight-loss manual had lost little weight. As you might expect, their cholesterol, HDL cholesterol, blood pressure, triglycerides, and other indicators of heart-disease risk stayed about the same. In contrast, the subjects who went through the weight-loss program had kept off an average 13 pounds by the end of 18 months (after having lost 22 pounds after 6 months). Heart disease risk factors improved temporarily in people who lost weight but then regained. In "successful" weight losers—defined as people who lost more than 10 pounds in the first 6 months and then stayed within 5 pounds of their new weight—changes were more lasting. Both HDL cholesterol levels and waist-to-hip ratios continued to improve over the 18-month study. The pattern of changes over time differed between men and women, but both sexes got about equal benefit from weight loss.

The value of this study and others like it is that it shows small weight losses can have good effects. All these people were at least 30 pounds overweight, and some were as much as 70 pounds too heavy. They lost on average only 22 pounds after 6 months and had regained an average of 8 pounds by 18 months. Even so, that amount of weight loss had good effects after 6 months. Benefits continued throughout the study for both men and women who kept off at least 10 pounds.

Studies like this one are great news. They show that you don't have to get down to an ideal weight to benefit from efforts to lose weight. In fact, just cutting back on calories may be enough to improve your glucose control and cut your risks of other diseases as well.

The Skinny on Chapter

▶ **Being overweight poses a big danger to your heart and blood vessels.**

▶ **Diabetes, obesity, high blood pressure, atherosclerosis, high triglyceride levels, low HDL levels, and high LDL levels tend to occur together in a heart-ravaging cluster.**

▶ **People who are overweight and people who lose a lot of weight quickly tend to get gallstones more often than other people.**

▶ **Overweight people are more likely to get some forms of cancer.**

▶ **Extra weight can put painful pressure on arthritic joints.**

▶ **Gout is more common in overweight people because they tend to have higher uric acid levels.**

▶ **People with diabetes who lose weight can control their glucose levels better.**

▶ **Getting health benefits from weight loss is not an all-or-nothing deal. Whatever you lose may help you, even if you're still far from your target weight.**

▶ **Losing just 10 or 20 pounds can have a big influence on your health. It can lower your glucose levels and your heart disease risk and make your joints more comfortable.**

▶ **Preventing weight gain will have positive effects on your health, and you may even live longer.**

The Best Way of Measuring Your Weight-Loss Progress Is by Tracking Your Health (Not Just Your Weight).

You probably hope that losing weight will bring about many good changes in your life. Another key to losing weight is that keeping track of your progress toward these changes is the best measure of how you're doing.

For example, you may want to have more energy, prevent complications, or lower your blood pressure. The number of pounds you've lost tells you a lot. But it doesn't tell you everything about your progress. Tracking your blood pressure, your glucose level, or how you feel fills out the picture. In fact, because good glucose control makes you feel better now and prevents complications later, your falling glucose level is a great measure of your progress.

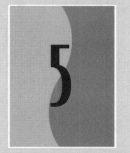

5

Your glucose level drops quickly as you lose weight, making it a good yardstick for success.

Glucose, Your First and Best Measure of Progress

I t might seem obvious that if your goal is to lose weight, the best way to track your success would be to keep track of how many pounds you've lost. Obvious—but not true.

Your real goals in losing weight have nothing to do with which numbers show up in the window of the scale and everything to do with feeling better and living longer. Because you have diabetes, losing weight can mean good changes in your life. Those changes, not arbitrary pounds, are what's important.

There are lots of ways to measure your weight-loss progress, but your best measure of weight-loss success is improvement in your diabetes. We'll look at this measure in this chapter, and Chapter 6 will suggest several other useful ways to track your progress.

WHY LOW GLUCOSE LEVELS ARE GOOD

Whether your doctor uses the homey, old-fashioned phrase "blood sugar" or leans to a scientific phrase such as "glucose level," you've been hearing about it since you were first diagnosed. You may be sick of measuring it, talking about it, and worrying about it. Why so much fuss about glucose?

Your glucose level signals how well your body is using the energy it gets from food. When a person eats carbohydrates, the body breaks down the complex molecules into a simple sugar molecule called glucose. In a person without diabetes, the glucose spurs the pancreas to release the hormone insulin into the blood. This insulin then tries to persuade cells to take in the glucose. Usually, the cells are glad to do so. They use energy from glucose to power their daily chores.

But in people with diabetes, things go wrong. In people with type 1 diabetes, the pancreas makes little or no insulin.

In people with type 2 diabetes, the cells resist the action of insulin and let glucose in slowly. Early on, the pancreas responds by pumping out more insulin. But as time goes by, the pancreas has a harder and harder time releasing enough, especially when glucose goes up after a meal.

Either way, the results are the same. Glucose builds up in the blood. These high levels can harm the eyes, kidneys, nerves, and blood vessels.

When you can keep your glucose levels close to normal, your body runs better. Your cells can do their jobs right. So you feel better and head off future problems.

THE EFFECTS OF WEIGHT LOSS ON DIABETES CONTROL

What Happens When People With Diabetes Lose Weight?

When you lose weight, you can expect your glucose level to fall and your diabetes control to improve. Your glucose level may even drop all the way to normal. This drop can have several good effects:

- If you have type 2 diabetes and are taking insulin, you may be able to cut back on your dose or switch to diabetes pills instead.

- If you are taking diabetes pills, you may be able to use a lower dose or stop taking pills altogether.

- If you stick with your new habits, you should get fewer complications in the future.

- If you have complications, they should progress more slowly.

- If you have been suffering symptoms of bad control such as blurry vision, tiredness, and needing to urinate often, these problems may clear up.

Why Your Doctor Needs to Know

You'll want your doctor to know about your weight-loss plan before you even start. The reason is that you may need changes in your insulin or diabetes pills right away. Glucose levels can fall quickly at the beginning of weight loss. Staying on the same treatment program as before may cause your glucose levels to fall too low. Low-glucose reactions (hypoglycemia) are especially a threat in the early stages of weight loss. To avoid reac-

APPETITE CONTROL LEADS TO DIABETES CONTROL

"I was so heavy at 15 months, I could hardly even sit up," says Melanie Cooper. She looks at photos of her baby self and sees "a little blimp."

She struggled with her weight for many years and tried a variety of weight-loss plans, with never more than temporary success. Hunger was her downfall. "I had never really been full," she says, except perhaps after stuffing herself at a banquet.

When she hit 335, her back began to pain her terribly. She went to her diabetes-care doctor, who found that Cooper's blood pressure was too high, as were her cholesterol and blood glucose levels. Her doctor sent her to a weight-loss clinic. Cooper started weight-loss drugs, which went to work on her appetite right away. "I would sit down and start eating, and I would have to eat less and less on my plate," she says. Suddenly—"like a snap of a finger"—she would find herself absolutely stuffed. "I had never experienced that before."

Being able to control her appetite let her finally lose weight. She dropped 75 pounds. She's now cut back from taking two blood pressure drugs to only one. Her cholesterol now hovers around 200 or 210. And her blood glucose level is normal.

tions, you'll want to test your glucose extra often at the start of your weight-loss program.

How Much Improvement Can You Expect?

A study in *Archives of Internal Medicine* in 1987 looked at how weight loss improved glucose levels. The study enrolled 114 overweight adults with type 2 diabetes in a weight-loss program for 10 to 16 weeks. The program consisted of learning to eat a reduced-calorie diet and being encouraged to become more active. Starting weight averaged 229 pounds for men and 208 pounds for women.

Glucose levels at the start averaged about 190 mg/dl. The average glycated hemoglobin (HbA_1) value was about 9.8%. (If you don't know what these numbers mean, see the box "Talking About Glucose Tests.") The results 1 year later showed that the more weight people lost, the better it was for their diabetes control.

The six people who had lost 30 pounds or more over that year had great results. They brought their fasting glucose levels down to an average of 109 mg/dl and their HbA_1 down to 7.1%. The 21 people who lost between 15 and 30 pounds brought their glucose down to 162 mg/dl and their HbA_1 to 8.7%. Most of these 27 people were able to cut back on their diabetes drugs.

This study shows that people don't need to lose all their excess weight to help their diabetes. Thirty pounds was enough to bring glucose way down, even though people who lost that much were still an average of 20% above their ideal weight. And 15 pounds had good effects, too, even though those people were still 43% overweight.

WHY TRACKING DIABETES CONTROL IS A GOOD IDEA

Keeping track of your glucose as you lose weight has several points in its favor:

- Falling glucose levels are meaningful. Lowering your glucose level directly improves your health.

- Falling glucose levels give you a quick reward. Glucose may start dropping within days of your starting a weight-loss plan. In contrast, it might take weeks to drop a dress size.

TALKING ABOUT GLUCOSE TESTS

I test my glucose level at home.
So why does my doctor test it at my visits?

Even trained lab professionals using the same lab tests can get different results. By testing you at your visits, your doctor gets a reading that can be compared with those of all the other clinic patients and with your own past and future results. Also, if your doctor's results are quite off from yours, it may signal a problem. For example, your meter may not be working right, or your technique may have gotten sloppy.

How do I know if my reading is good?

Glucose in your doctor's test and in your home meter is measured in milligrams per deciliter (mg/dl). A normal reading is defined as one that falls between 70 and 110 mg/dl when someone hasn't eaten in several hours.

   Just because this range is normal does not mean it's the best goal for everyone with diabetes. When people have very high glucose levels (greater than 200 mg/dl), their goal may be set between 110 and 140 mg/dl—a big improvement.

My doctor also does a glycated hemoglobin test. What's that?

When blood glucose levels are high, glucose molecules grab onto proteins and don't let go. Glycated hemoglobin tests measure the percentage of hemoglobin molecules that have glucose molecules stuck to them. Red blood cells—the cells that contain hemoglobin—live 3 to 4 months. So the glycated hemoglobin test gives a picture of what your control has been like on average during that time.

   One of the most common glycated hemoglobin tests measures glucose attached to one specific kind of hemoglobin, called hemoglobin A_1. You'll often see this test abbreviated as HbA_{1c} or HbA1c.

Continued

TALKING ABOUT GLUCOSE TESTS *Continued*

In a person without diabetes, about 5% of hemoglobin molecules have glucose attached. But different labs use different methods of measuring glycated hemoglobin, and they give different results. So you'll have to ask your doctor what your values mean.

At my last doctor's visit, I had a high glucose level, but my HbA$_{1c}$ was good. Why didn't the results agree?

A blood glucose test is like a snapshot. It shows your glucose at one instant in time. What you've eaten, how active you've been, and when you've taken any diabetes drugs all can affect it. And it does not tell you what's going on the rest of the time.

If you keep records of your results from home testing, they fill in some of the gaps. They can show the various ups and downs your glucose goes through while you're awake. They can also reveal possible problems that need looking into—for example, that your glucose level stays high long after you eat pizza or that your first glucose reading on Sunday mornings is always low.

But even if you tested your blood glucose 40 times a day (ouch!), you couldn't fill in all the gaps. Here's where the HbA$_{1c}$ can help. Because it's an average, it reflects all your glucose levels. It won't be thrown off just because you had to run for the bus this morning. It gives a picture of your overall control.

I'd like to track my long-term glucose levels at home and not have to wait for my doctor's visit to find out how I'm doing. Isn't there something I can do?

An at-home test for glycated fructosamine was approved in December 1997. Like hemoglobin, other proteins in the blood, such as albumin, can get glucoses stuck to them. "Fructosamine" is the name given to these protein-glucose combo molecules. The new fructosamine test measures the level of fructosamine in the blood.

Fructosamine has a shorter life than the hemoglobin protein. So the fructosamine test reveals average control over a shorter time: the

TALKING ABOUT GLUCOSE TESTS *Continued*

past 2 to 3 weeks. Testing as often as your doctor suggests can let you know whether changes you've made recently are helping or hurting your glucose control.

In the fructosamine test, levels less than 310 micromoles per liter (µmol/l) show good control. Levels greater than 380 µmol/l show poor control.

- Falling glucose levels show true success in managing your diabetes. Weight can bounce up and down. It may stabilize before you're ready to stop losing weight. But your glucose level tells you whether you have met one of your main goals: improving your health.

Your glucose is not the only measure of how your diabetes is doing. You can track improvement in your diabetes in several other areas:

- Are you able to use a lower dose of insulin to keep the same good level of control?

- Is a lower dose of diabetes pills helping your glucose to stay close to normal?

- Is your vision less blurry? (If better glucose control does not get rid of all the blurriness, see your eye doctor. You might need new glasses. Or you may have the start of diabetic eye disease, and early treatment will help you keep the best vision.)

- Do you have more energy?

- Are cuts and sores healing more quickly?

- Does your skin itch less?

Chapter 6 contains some tables you can copy to keep track of your progress in these and other areas.

The Skinny on Chapter

5

- ▶ Diabetes treatments are aimed at reducing glucose levels.
- ▶ This focus on glucose levels makes sense because in people with diabetes, keeping glucose levels as close to normal as possible protects organs from damage.
- ▶ Your body converts carbohydrates into glucose, a kind of sugar.
- ▶ The pancreas produces insulin, which helps glucose enter cells.
- ▶ Losing even a small percentage of your weight can bring your glucose levels down quite a bit—sometimes quickly.
- ▶ Some people's glucose levels return to the normal range after weight loss.
- ▶ Because weight loss improves glucose control, it's vital to adjust the amount of diabetes drug (and sometimes the kind, as well) to avoid low-blood-glucose reactions.

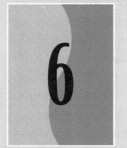

6

Other Measures of Progress

You have many choices for tracking how well you're doing in your weight-loss efforts.

One of the perks of being a tyrant is having great minds at your command. Hiero II, tyrant of the Greek colony of Syracuse, was luckier than most. His subjects included one of the greatest scientists of all time, Archimedes. So, according to legend, when Hiero wanted to find out whether a crown was pure gold, he knew whom to ask.

Archimedes puzzled over his assignment for a while. Then inspiration struck him as he stepped into his bath. The water overflowed, and the overjoyed Archimedes ran naked through the city shouting, "Eureka!" (Greek for "I have found it!").

What had he found? A way to measure an object's density by submerging it in water. Archimedes put Hiero's crown in a container of water and measured how much water it displaced. He also put pure gold (an amount that weighed the same in air as the crown) in water. If the crown were also pure gold, both objects would be equally dense and so would displace an equal amount of water. But Hiero's crown caused more water to overflow. So Archimedes knew that the crown could not be pure gold, but must contain a less-dense metal that gave it a greater volume.

Archimedes' method for measuring densities is, even today, the best way to find out how much fat you have and how much you are losing in your weight-loss program. But this method is awkward and requires special equipment. So this chapter will also tell you about some of the other ways you can follow your progress. And to help you track how you're doing, Tables 6-1, 6-2, 6-3, and 6-4 provide forms that you can photocopy. (Figures 6-1, 6-2, 6-3, and 6-4 show filled-out examples.) And if a visual record is more your style, Figure 6-5 is a blank graph that you can copy and use to chart your weight changes. Over the weeks, a graph can really help you to see your weight dropping and can let you know when you're leveling off.

POUNDS LOST

The best reason to step on the bathroom scale is that weighing is a simple, quick way to get an idea how you are doing. Excess body weight is linked to many health problems. So weighing yourself can give you an idea of changes you can expect in your blood pressure, cholesterol levels, triglyceride levels, and other measures discussed later in this chapter.

Some scientists believe you should weigh yourself often. Weights do vary from day to day. Some people's weight varies a lot. Women's weights tend to go up and down in sync with their menstrual cycle. Changes in the amount of water in the body lead to weight being a bit higher just before one's period.

By measuring every day, at least at first, you will learn your pattern. Then you will know better what to make of a 2- or 3-pound change. It might be a sign of change in the right (or wrong!) direction. Or it might just be the amount you'd expect to vary over a few weeks.

But some doctors believe that weighing once a week or less is plenty. They object to using lost pounds as a measure of success for several reasons:

- Lost pounds as guideposts mislead people into focusing on getting slim, instead of on getting healthy. Eating right and exercising are then viewed as means to the goal of slimness, rather than as worthwhile goals themselves.

- The good effects of losing 10 pounds or 20 pounds depend in part on how tall you are.

- Small amounts of weight loss can have good effects on many aspects of your life. If you measure success in pounds, losing 10% of your weight may seem a failure. But measured in health improvements, losing 10% of your weight may be a grand success.

- Your scale can't distinguish lost muscle pounds from lost fat pounds. But only the fat pounds are harmful.

No matter how often you weigh yourself, what you'll probably see is that weight tends to come off faster at first. Weight lost at the start consists mainly of water and carbohydrates in temporary storage. After a while, you may taper off to losing a pound or two a week. The content of the pounds you lose shifts to include more fat. This slowing down of weight loss is normal and no reason to become discouraged. Even though you're losing less weight, you're burning off the pounds that matter—fat pounds. Steady progress downward is what's important.

MEASURES OF OVERALL FATNESS

Two people can be the same height and weight, yet have very different amounts of fat. Think of a large-boned person who lifts weights regularly vs. a small-boned person who spends a lot of time on the couch. The first person has more muscle and bone and less fat than the second. This example shows why your weight alone cannot tell you whether you've reached a good size or still have too much fat.

Body Mass Index

You learned about body mass index (BMI) in Chapter 1 as a way to get a quick idea of whether your weight is right or not. Table 1-1 lists BMIs for a wide range of heights and weights. Because BMIs are often used to figure your risk of diseases related to overweight, tracking your BMI is a good way to see how your health is improving. BMIs between 20 and 25 are thought to be healthiest.

As people get older, they tend to lose lean tissue, and they tend to put on fat. Although people usually gain a little weight until about age 60,

TABLE 6-1

Daily Record for the Month of _____

Measurement	1	2	3	4	5	6	7	8	9	10	11	12	13	14	15
Weight															
Fasting glucose level															
Landmarks															
Exercised?															
Calories eaten															

	16	17	18	19	20	21	22	23	24	25	26	27	28	29	30	31
Weight																
Fasting glucose level																
Landmarks																
Exercised?																
Calories eaten																

FIGURE 6-1

Sample Daily Record

Measurement	1	2	3	4	5	6	7	8	9	10	11	12	13	14	15
Weight	148	147	148	147	147	147	140	150	150	151	160	149	149	147	148
Fasting glucose level	130	125	120	130	125	130	140	150	150	150	130	125	130	125	115
Cooked ruist	✓	✓	✓	✓	✓	✓					✓	✓	✓	✓	✓
Landmarks made it to post office on ...											✗				
Exercised? walked (min)	30	45		20	21	39				35	60	30	30	45	
Calories eaten	1500				1600						1200	1100	1200	1200	1360

	16	17	18	19	20	21	22	23	24	25	26	27	28	29	30	31
Weight	146	147	146	145	144	143	144	144 (forget to weigh)	143	142	142	141	141	141	141	140
Fasting glucose level	90	100	115	125	115	110	130	120	135	120	115	120	115	120	130	110
Cooked lmurfat	✓	✓		✓		✓	✓	✓	✓	✓	✓	✓	✓	✓	✓	✓
Landmarks below a BMI of 25					✗											
Exercised? walked (min)		30		41	50	22	25	35			42	50	41	30	30	36
Calories eaten				1400							1300	1400				

TABLE 6-2

Quarterly Record for Doctor's Visits in the Year _____

Measurement		Date of doctor's visit			
Name	**Normal value**				
	< means less than > means greater than				
Weight					
BMI	<25				
HbA1c					
Blood pressure	<140/90 mmHg				
Total cholesterol	<200 mg/dl				
LDL cholesterol	<130 mg/dl				
HDL cholesterol	>35 mg/dl				
Triglycerides	<160 mg/dl				

FIGURE 6-2

Sample Quarterly Record

Measurement		Date of doctor's visit			
Name	Normal value	2/4	5/19	8/8	11/18
	< means less than > means greater than				
Weight	<142 lb.	160	145	131	142
BMI	<25	28.4	25.7	23.3	25.2
HbA1c Westin Labs ref. range	<7.5%	9%	8%	7.5%	7.8%
Blood pressure	<140/90 mmHg	150/90	didn't measure	120/80	125/80
Total cholesterol	<200 mg/dl	250	⟲	180	didn't measure
LDL cholesterol	<130 mg/dl	190	⟲	130	⟲
HDL cholesterol	>35 mg/dl	25	⟲	35	⟲
Triglycerides	<160 mg/dl	60	⟲	35	⟲

TABLE 6-3

Record for the Year _____

Measurement	Jan 1	Feb 1	Mar 1	Apr 1	May 1	Jun 1	Jul 1	Aug 1	Sep 1	Oct 1	Nov 1	Dec 1
Weight												
BMI												
Waist												
Hip												
Waist-to-hip ratio												
Blood pressure												
Insulin dose												
Diabetes pill dose												

FIGURE 6-3

Sample Yearly Record

Measurement	Jan 1	Feb 1	Mar 1	Apr 1	May 1	Jun 1	Jul 1	Aug 1	Sep 1	Oct 1	Nov 1	Dec 1
Weight	165	155	150	145	140	135	130	130	130	140	145	140
BMI	29.3	27.5	26.6	25.7	24.9	24.0	23.1	23.1	23.1	24.9	25.7	24.9
Waist	35	33	32	31	31	30	29	29	29½	30	31	31
Hip	42	41	41	41	40	39	39	39	40	40	40	40
Waist-to-hip ratio	0.83	0.80	0.78	0.76	0.76	0.77	0.74	0.74	0.74	0.75	0.78	0.78
Blood pressure	150/90	145/90	140/85	130/80	110/70	120/60	115/80	120/80	115/70	130/80	120/80	120/80
Insulin dose	—	—	—	—	—	—	—	—	—	—	—	—
Diabetes pill dose metformin	2500 mg	2000 mg	2000 mg	2000 mg	1500 mg	1500 mg	1500 mg	—	—	—	—	—

TABLE 6-4

Sample Contract with Yourself

Terms	
Who is making the contract?	
How long will this contract last?	
What is the goal?	
How often?	
How long each time?	
When?	
Signature	
Date	
Witness	

FIGURE 6-4

Sample Contract

Terms	
Who is making the contract?	Jane Doerr
How long will this contract last?	April 1 – June 1
What is the goal?	I will buy at least one low-fat cookbook by April 1. I will cook meals with <25% of calories from fat.
How often?	6 days a week
How long each time?	N/A
When?	Supper
Signature	Jane Doerr
Date	3-25-97
Witness	Phil T. Smith

FIGURE 6-5

A Record of Your Weight for the Month of _____

On the first day of the month, write your weight on the line next to the heavy horizontal bar. On each day after that, make an x where your weight falls that day. For example, if you start the month weighing 200 pounds and on the 10th you weigh 205, you would put an x where the vertical line marked "10" crosses the horizontal line labeled "+5." (If you prefer, you can label the horizontal lines each month. Each line stands for 1 pound.)

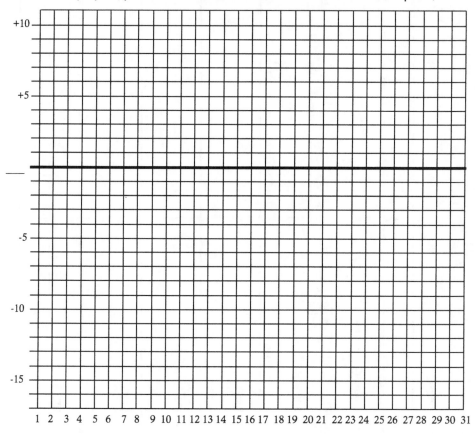

the effects on weight of adding fat and losing lean tissue sometimes cancel each other out. If there is no weight gain, but only a change in the relative amounts of fat and muscle, then BMI may stay the same even though the person is in truth becoming fatter. So some scientists suggest that BMI is less useful as a measure of fatness in older people. As a result, some suggest that older people need their own BMI table with different cutoffs.

Percentage Body Fat

The most valuable indicator of how fat you are is the percentage of your tissues that are fat. In general, men should be less than 25% fat, and women should be less than 40% fat.

Your doctor or a local health club may have equipment that can estimate your fat. (See the box "Methods of Measuring Fat.")

MEASURES OF ABDOMINAL FAT

Some people are evenly fat all over. Some people's fat clusters around their middle, giving them an apple shape. And some people's fat deposits on the hips and thighs, giving them a pear shape.

As you learned in Chapter 2, fat on the abdomen is thought to be particularly risky for the heart and blood vessels. Evenly distributed fat and fat on the hips and thighs might cause fewer health problems. So your shape may provide extra clues to your health.

The effects of weight loss on body shape are in dispute. Some studies find that losing weight causes the body to become a little more pear-like; others find no change in shape; and many other studies find that people lose the most fat from where they have the most fat—that is, people who are apple-like may lose more waist inches than pear-like people do.

These three sets of results sound contradictory, but may not be. If people do lose fat from their fattest areas, then whether or not a study finds that people become more pear-like might depend on where the subjects had the most fat to start with. It's also possible that whether weight losers become more pear-shaped depends on how much exercise they do.

In any case, losing weight will reduce the fat on your abdomen and elsewhere and help your health. Two ways to track these changes are the waist measurement and the waist-to-hip ratio.

METHODS OF MEASURING FAT

Several methods of measuring your percentage of body fat are fairly quick, simple, cheap, and safe. None of these is particularly accurate for detecting small changes. Still, unless you live in a very small town, it's easy to find a health club, health fair (held at your company or at the mall, for instance), or weight-loss clinic that can perform at least one of these measures on you. These simple, safe measures are:

- Bioelectric impedance analysis, in which your fat is measured by voltage differences between your fat and lean tissues (home bioelectric impedance analyzers are starting to become available)

- Skin-fold measurement, in which your fat is estimated from the thickness of the fat lying right under your skin

- Hydrostatic weighing (Archimedes' method), in which your fat is estimated by the water overflow from a tank (just like Hiero's crown)

- Near-infrared interactance, a controversial method in which fat is detected by shining a light through your arm

- Ultrasound, in which fat is mapped with sound waves, just as ships map the sea floor by bouncing sound off it

Near-infrared interactance is thought to be fairly error-prone. Underwater weighing is considered the most accurate of these five methods. Still, none of them are 100% reliable, for at least three reasons:

METHODS OF MEASURING FAT *Continued*

- Except for ultrasound, these methods get at your fat content indirectly. First, something other than fat is measured. Then, that measurement is translated into fat percentage by an equation that assumes you are typical. But you may have larger muscles than average, or you may be dehydrated. Bioelectic impedance analysis, skin-fold measurements, and near-infrared interactance tend to give too low a fat percentage in people who are overweight. And bioelectric impedance gives inaccurate results for people with diabetes unless their glucose is under tight control.

- Technique matters. With skin folds, for example, both the calipers and the technician wielding them can affect the result. Ultrasound is hard to perform the same way every time. Also, there are a variety of equations for converting measurements to fat. Different equations do not always give the same answers.

- Often, estimation equations were developed with young white subjects. But people of different ages and races sometimes differ biologically. For example, blacks tend to have denser bones than whites, and older people tend not to carry half their fat right under their skin as younger people do. So unless the right conversion equation is used correctly, the result may be off.

There are several ways to get a more accurate measurement of your fat (at least in some parts of your body). But these require costly, awkward tests that are used mostly for research studies on fat. Like ultrasound, these tests are based on imaging methods—that is, they involve sending waves of some kind through your body and creating a picture of your fat. Three of these methods that you may hear about are computed tomography, dual-energy X-ray absorptiometry (which is becoming more available), and magnetic resonance imaging.

Of course, neither method gives a view inside the body. If someone has a large waist, it may be due to extra fat padding around his or her internal organs. Or it may be due to extra fat under the skin. (In most people, it's due to extra fat in both places.) Is the location of fat important? Some scientists believe fat around the organs may be riskier than fat under the skin. There's still a lot to be learned about the dangers of where you carry your fat.

Men and women have different patterns of putting on fat. So do younger people and older people. And it appears people of different races may also differ in fat deposition. More research is needed to figure out how these patterns of putting on fat affect health and what the best ways to measure abdominal fat in different people are.

Waist Measurement

Waist measurement (circumference) alone seems a skimpy piece of data by which to measure your success. It's just one number that doesn't take into account whether you're tall or short, an apple or a pear. But in fact, waist measurement seems to be a good marker both for fat on the abdomen and for total fat in the body—possibly better than waist-to-hip ratio. It may also be a better marker for heart disease risk. So if you don't have a calculator, keeping track of your waist measurement alone saves you from doing a lot of math by hand and may be just as useful.

In fact, you may already be doing a version of this test. Do you have a skirt or pair of pants that you try on regularly to see how it fits? This is one way to monitor whether your waist size is increasing or decreasing.

There are no generally accepted standards for what a healthy waist measurement is. One research group found that a waist size larger than 39 inches is unhealthy for whites and suggested that white men and women should try to reduce their waists below this figure. Another group also found that a waist under 39 inches meant healthier insulin and glucose levels in obese women of unspecified race. But a different group, apparently working with white subjects, suggested a limit of 37 inches for men and 31 inches in women was healthiest.

Waist-to-Hip Ratio

The waist-to-hip ratio is the measure doctors use most often to find out abdominal fat. In Chapter 2, you learned how to figure out your waist-to-hip ratio. The best ratio for women is less than 0.8. The best ratio for men is less than 1.0.

As people age, their bodies change in many ways. Skin and muscles become less firm, and water content may change. Because of these changes, the waist-to-hip ratio may not be as good a measure of body fat in older people.

The waist-to-hip ratio is not a risk factor for heart disease itself. Rather, it reflects what heart disease risk factors are present. By tracking your waist-to-hip ratio at home, you get a simple, single-number estimate of your burden of risks. A high ratio also serves as an alert to people who aren't overweight that they may still have more fat buildup on their abdomens than is healthy.

MAKING THE CHOICE TO LIVE

Boom, boom, boom. Life came down hard on Diego Garcia in 1993. His chest hurt, and he had to have surgery on his blood vessels (angioplasty). "At that time, I stopped smoking, and that's when I started to pick up the weight," he says. The 50 new pounds he gained pressed terribly on his arthritic hip. "I just couldn't move anymore. And between the pain in my hip, which was unbearable, and the weight, I was killing myself," he says. He was on the road to needing a hip replacement. But the doctors told him, "We won't touch you unless you lose at least 50 pounds."

Garcia chose to live. He's now down to 220 pounds (from 311). (You'll read more about how he did it in Chapter 7.) He recently had his hip replaced, and the new hip is working perfectly. His blood glucose has dropped into the normal range, and so has his blood pressure. His life has improved along with his health.

"I've got a 6-year-old son, and I like to do things with him," says Garcia. "But with my hip being so bad and weighing so much, I couldn't even get on a bike a year and a half, 2 years ago." Now he can't wait. "When it gets warm, I'm going to jump on that bike and do some riding!"

MEASURES OF QUALITY OF LIFE

Excess weight can play havoc with people's lives. When you lose weight, many aspects of your life may get better. Here are some ideas for aspects you may wish to track:

- How much money you spend on diabetes drugs (insulin or pills) or blood pressure drugs

- How many blocks you can walk or steps you can climb

- How long it takes to walk a certain distance, such as to the store or dry cleaners

- How well you sleep at night

- When you hit important firsts: the first time you fit into a seat at a movie theater, the first time you sleep through the night, the first time you buy an outfit that's not a plus size, or the first time you can ride a bicycle

MEASURES OF HEALTH IMPROVEMENT

People who are overweight often have weight-related health problems. In Chapter 5, you read about the benefits of tracking changes in your diabetes. If you have other weight-related problems, you may wish to monitor their improvement as well.

Blood Pressure

Obesity and high blood pressure go hand in hand. When you go on a weight-loss program, you can be pretty sure your blood pressure will improve. Studies show that blood pressure drops occur within the first 2 or 3 weeks. Losing about 10 pounds can bring about good changes. Losing more weight helps even more. Also, high blood pressure drugs have many side effects. Losing weight allows some people to cut back or even stop taking these drugs.

If you have a blood pressure device or have some other way to measure your pressure often, blood pressure is a good number to track.

TALKING ABOUT BLOOD PRESSURE READINGS

Why do blood pressure measurements have two numbers?

The first number is called the systolic pressure. It tells the force with which your blood travels through your arteries when your heart squeezes. The second number is called the diastolic pressure. It tells the force of your blood when your heart is relaxed. Blood pressures are given in millimeters of mercury (mmHg).

How do I know whether my blood pressure is too high?

High blood pressure is defined as a reading higher than 140/90 mmHg. Average normal blood pressure is defined as 120/80 mmHg.

Only one of my numbers is too high. Do I have high blood pressure or not?

You may. Having only one number be too high, especially the diastolic pressure, can still be risky for your heart and brain.

My friend said she had "white-coat hypertension." What's that?

Some people have high blood pressure (hypertension) only when they're at the doctor's office. Researchers are unsure whether this indicates a health problem or whether these people just get jittery around doctors.

Are there any other times when a person whose blood pressure is fine may have a too-high reading?

A falsely high blood pressure can also result from bad technique (for example, putting the cuff on wrong), smoking, a full bladder, or even seeing a look of worry on the doctor's face.

Because blood pressure falls quickly at the start of a weight-loss program, you get a reward for your efforts right away. (See the box "Spotlight on Research: Losing Weight Lowers Blood Pressure.")

Other Health Improvements

You may have other health problems that you hope will improve with weight loss. You might want to track:

- Total cholesterol level

- LDL ("bad") cholesterol level

- HDL ("good") cholesterol level

- Triglyceride level

- Severity of arthritis pain (for example, on a scale of 1 to 10)

A CONTRACT WITH YOURSELF

Some people find the best way to set goals and follow their progress is to draw up a contract.

Of course, a contract with yourself is not a legal document. You will not be able to sue yourself for nonperformance if you don't live up to it! But such a contract does help you set clear goals and commit to them.

A good contract with yourself has several elements:

- The dates to which it applies—for example, "now until Christmas"

- A precise definition of what you will do—for example, "I will take brisk walks"

- A minimum goal for how often you will do each activity—for example, "5 days a week"

- A minimum goal for how long you will do each activity, if appropriate—for example, "30 minutes at a time"

SPOTLIGHT ON RESEARCH

Losing Weight Lowers Blood Pressure

Phase II of the Trials of Hypertension Prevention is one of many studies that show the good effects of weight loss on blood pressure. This study, published in the *Archives of Internal Medicine* in 1997, looked at the effects of weight loss and sodium restriction on high blood pressure. (Sodium from salt raises blood pressure in some people.) The subjects were 2,382 overweight people between the ages of 30 and 54. None had diabetes. All had a diastolic blood pressure of 83 to 89 mmHg, and their systolic pressures were less than 140 mmHg. (If you don't know what these numbers mean, see the box "Talking About Blood Pressure Readings.") These numbers are on the high end of normal, suggesting that these people were at risk of one day getting high blood pressure.

One-quarter of the people received only the care they otherwise would have. Another quarter received instructions for lowering their salt intake. A third quarter received counseling about losing weight. And a final group worked on both eating less salt and losing weight.

After 6 months, people in the two groups that tried to lose weight had dropped roughly 9 pounds. People in the two low-salt groups had cut their salt intake somewhat. Both treatments had an effect on blood pressure. Compared with the group that received usual care, the people in the other groups lowered their systolic pressures by 3 to 4 mmHg and their diastolic pressures by 1.6 to 2.8 mmHg. To scientists' surprise, losing weight lowered blood pressure better than cutting salt.

Over the next 3 to 4 years, blood pressures of the people in the three treatment groups went up some. As you might guess, so did their weight and salt intake. Still, their blood pressures did not return to the pre-study levels.

A few points of blood pressure improvement may not sound like much. But other studies have found that drops of as little as 2 mmHg can lower stroke and heart disease risks.

This study shows that losing weight and cutting salt can both lower blood pressure. But losing weight works a good deal better.

■ A goal for when you will do each activity—for example, "before breakfast"

Sign and date your contract. Also have a friend or relative sign your contract. These acts strengthen your commitment to your goal. Your witness will also know what you are doing and can offer support and help (and any needed nagging). Once you have a clear goal, you can keep track of it with whatever other measures of success you are monitoring.

Table 6-4 and Figure 6-4 show a sample contract form.

The Skinny on Chapter

6

► Archimedes, perhaps the inventor of streaking, figured out 2,200 years ago how to measure an object's density by putting it in water. This method is the best way to estimate a person's fat content.

► The number of pounds you've lost is an easy way to measure your progress. But it gives little information about how much your life is improving.

► Body mass index is a simple clue to whether you are the right size for your height.

► Your percentage of body fat is the best indicator of how fat you are.

► Fat around the internal organs may be more dangerous than fat under the skin.

► Two ways of tracking shape changes are the waist measurement and the waist-to-hip ratio.

► The waist-to-hip ratio has been much studied. Doctors know that higher values are linked to heart disease and diabetes complications.

► Keeping track of simple pleasures of life such as the ability to do all your grocery shopping without taking a rest break can help you see your progress.

► High blood pressure is dangerous, and blood pressure usually rises and falls with weight. So when you see your blood pressure fall, you know that your chance of death is also falling.

► You may also wish to track other health problems related to overweight.

A Healthful, Low-Calorie Diet Is the Only Good Way to Take Off Pounds.

3

A typical bookstore has shelves and shelves of weight-loss books. Magazine covers blare news about weight loss in every grocery store check-out lane. All sorts of diets get passed along by word of mouth. But in truth, there's only one good, scientifically proven way to lose weight. That's to eat fewer calories than you burn. These chapters will lay out for you the most up-to-date research on what a good diet is and guide you in improving your own. Most important, these chapters aim to convince you that healthful food choices are not dull or weird or unpleasant. Rather, you can eat tasty, filling meals while losing weight.

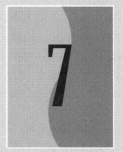

CHAPTER

7

The best diet for someone who has diabetes or who is trying to lose weight is much like the best diet for anyone— plenty of fruits, vegetables, and grains, with relatively few calories from fat.

Choosing Your Diet

Have you ever happened on some old magazines and riffled through them? The odd, impractical outfits jump off the page. Women cleaning house in high heels! Men wearing undershirts under their shirts, even in the middle of July! College students decked out in beanies!

Food plans from years ago seem odd and impractical now, too. If you've had diabetes for awhile, you remember when sugar was a no-no. Doctors told people with diabetes to avoid eating sugar. At the same time, food companies were adding sugar to all sorts of food, including salty crackers. As a result, people with diabetes couldn't eat the same diet as the rest of society. People trying to lose weight, who were sometimes told to limit their carbohydrates, had the same problem.

Today, the situation is quite different. A good diet is a good diet. There's not much difference between what people with diabetes should eat for good glucose control, what overweight people should eat for weight loss, and what people in general should eat for best health.

This chapter will describe what scientists today consider the best diet for Americans. Chapters 8, 9, and 10 will show you how to put these guidelines into practice in your own life.

THE BEST FOOD PLAN

Every few years, the U.S. Department of Agriculture and the U.S. Department of Health and Human Services ask scientists to review studies on the relationships among weight, diet, and health. The 1995 *Dietary Guidelines for Americans* contain the advice of the most recent expert panel. The guidelines in part explain what scientists believe to be the best diet for people above the age of 2.

One new feature of the 1995 guidelines is a shift from stressing weight loss to stressing weight maintenance. Don't let this shift fool you into thinking that being overweight is not as bad as previously thought! The expert panel saw how hard it can be to lose weight and decided that the old suggestion to lose weight was not practical for everyone. But staying at the same weight is another matter. It's doable for most people. Weight maintenance may keep your weight-related problems from getting worse. And for your friends and relatives who are not overweight, preventing weight gain may save them from the weight-related problems you've suffered.

Despite the new stress on weight maintenance, the *Dietary Guidelines for Americans* still encourage people who are overweight to lose weight. They point out that weight loss of 5% to 10% can improve high blood pressure and diabetes.

The Food Guide Pyramid

The four food groups have gone the way of the raccoon coat and poodle skirt. Today's guide to good eating—for everyone, including people with diabetes—is the Food Guide Pyramid. The pyramid (Figure 7-1) divides foods into five groups and shows the role each group should play in the diet.

The Food Guide Pyramid's serving sizes are given mostly in standard kitchen measurements, such as ounces and cups. If you do not have much cooking experience, you may have no idea how much a cup of lettuce or an ounce of cereal is. The best way to learn is to measure out servings at first. In fact, dietitians suggest that doing so can help everyone who is counting servings as part of a diabetes diet. After a short time of weighing and measuring your food, you will have a good idea of just how big each serving size is.

FIGURE 7-1

The USDA Food Guide Pyramid

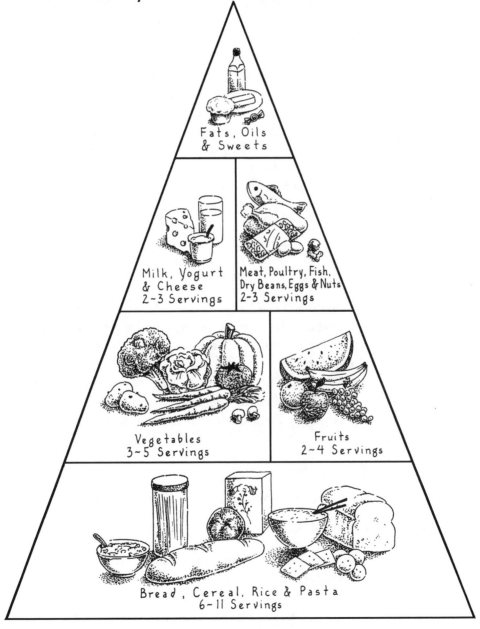

According to the Food Guide Pyramid, plant foods—grains, vegetables, and fruits—should make up most of the diet. You'll see that it suggests eating 11 to 20 servings of plant foods a day, but only 4 to 6 servings of animal foods. The range is large because different people need different amounts of food. The lower suggested servings are suitable for people who are cutting calories to lose weight.

The Grain Products Group. The foods at the bottom of the pyramid should form the base of the diet. These important foods are the grains. The Grain Products Group includes both grains in their simplest form (for example, rice, barley, and oats) and prepared grains (such as bread, breakfast cereal, and noodles). The Food Guide Pyramid suggests that Americans eat 6 to 11 servings of grains every day. (For people who are trying to cut calories and lose weight, 6 to 8 servings may be a good target.) Examples of one serving are:

- 1 slice of bread

- 1 ounce of cereal

- 1/2 cup of cooked cereal, rice, or pasta

For people with diabetes who base their diet on the Exchange Lists of the American Diabetes Association (ADA) and The American Dietetic Association, one serving from the Grain Products Group usually equals one Starch Exchange.

The Vegetable Group. The Vegetable Group contains all kinds of fresh vegetables, vegetable juices, and dried beans and peas. The Food Guide Pyramid suggests eating 3 to 5 servings a day from this group. One serving means:

- 1 cup of raw leafy vegetables

- 1/2 cup of other vegetables (cooked or chopped)

- 3/4 cup of vegetable juice

One serving from the Vegetable Group usually equals either 1 ADA Starch Exchange or 1/2 to 1 1/2 ADA Vegetable Exchanges.

Vegetables vary a lot in their calories. Low-calorie ones include greens (spinach, mustard greens, leaf lettuces, and turnip greens), peppers, green beans, celery, summer squashes, and cabbage-family vegetables (which include broccoli and cauliflower).

The Fruit Group. You can easily guess what foods are in the Fruit Group: fruits. Two to 4 servings each day from the Fruit Group is best. One serving is:

- 1 medium apple, banana, or orange

- 1/2 cup chopped, cooked, or canned fruit

- 3/4 cup of fruit juice

One serving from the Fruit Group equals roughly one Fruit Exchange. Low-calorie fruits include berries (blackberries, blueberries, currants, raspberries, and strawberries), grapefruit, grapes, apricots, peaches, plums, oranges, and watermelon.

The Milk Group. Milk, cheese, and yogurt are among the foods in the Milk Group. The Food Guide Pyramid suggests 2 to 3 servings from this group each day. Examples of one serving are:

- 1 cup of milk

- 1 cup of yogurt

- 1 1/2 ounces of regular cheese

- 2 ounces of processed cheese

One Milk Group serving of milk or yogurt equals 1 ADA Milk Exchange. One Milk Group serving of cheese equals 1 1/2 to 2 ADA Meat Exchanges.

Milk products also vary greatly in calories. Switching from drinking three glasses of regular milk a day to drinking three glasses of skim milk would save you 192 calories if you made no other changes in your diet.

The Meat and Beans Group. The Meat and Beans Group contains a wide variety of high-protein foods: meat (from mammals, birds, reptiles, or fish), cooked dried beans, eggs, and nuts.

Dried beans, peas, and lentils are members of both this group and the Vegetable Group. The Food Guide Pyramid says to count them as servings from one or the other but not both at the same time.

Two to 3 servings of this group each day are best. Serving sizes for the Meat and Beans Group are less specific than those for the other groups. They are best understood compared with the Meat Exchanges. One ADA Meat Exchange equals 1 ounce of cheese, chicken, fish, shellfish, game, lamb, veal, pork, or beef; one egg; or two egg whites. (Note that in the Exchange system, cheese can count as either a Meat Exchange or a Milk Exchange, but in the Food Guide Pyramid, cheese belongs only to the Milk Group.) One serving from the Food Guide Pyramid's Meat and Beans Group equals 2 to 3 Meat Exchanges.

Fats, Oils, and Sweets. At the top of the Food Guide Pyramid, taking up the least space of all, are the leftover foods that don't fit into any of the food groups: fats, oils, and sweets. The Food Guide Pyramid suggests that people choose sparingly from this group. In the Exchange Lists, many of these foods count as Other Carbohydrates Exchanges or Fat Exchanges.

Alcohol. Because the *Dietary Guidelines for Americans* are out of sync with the ADA guidelines for alcohol, this book will give you the latter instead. ADA suggests that men with diabetes have no more than two drinks a day and women with diabetes, no more than one. One drink means 12 ounces of beer, 5 ounces of wine, or 1 1/2 ounces of distilled spirits. For both people on insulin and those who take diabetes pills, alcohol should always be drunk with a meal, not by itself.

Alcohol is high in calories. A can of regular beer has 150 calories, which can be a tenth or more of the daily calorie budget for someone trying to lose weight. ADA suggests that people who count Exchanges or count calories should treat one alcoholic drink as 2 Fat Exchanges.

Other Components of a Good Diet. The *Dietary Guidelines for Americans* also say that Americans should choose a varied diet with plenty of fiber, vitamins, and minerals, including calcium. A good diet is also low in fats and cholesterol, with only moderate amounts of salt and sugar. The guidelines warn that foods with sugar substitutes are not always lower in calories than foods with sugar. Eating a diet based on the Food Guide Pyramid is a big step toward these goals.

Diets for Pregnant Women

If you are pregnant, eating a nutritious diet is extra important. But so is eating in a way that keeps your glucose levels controlled. Balancing these

CHANGING FOOD HABITS

Diego Garcia was always leery of diets that focused on salads. "I said, if I was going to be miserable, forget it." He also shied away from fad diets. His ex-wife once tried a high-protein liquid diet that was imbalanced, and she almost died.

But when he went to a weight-loss center, it pointed him in a different direction: learning more about healthy foods. As a result, says Garcia, "I've become more attuned to fat." He has also changed his eating habits. "A lot of the meat that I eat at home is turkey," he says. "I would never touch skim milk [before]. I thought that it was just white water, to be honest with you. And now I drink skim milk." And he and his family now buy and eat many fat-free products.

Changing his eating habits has been wrenching for Garcia because eating and food have always been important parts of family life. But his family is also the reason he's stuck with his changes. "We had a child later in life, in our 40s," he says. Now he wants to see that son grow up.

two goals can be tricky. And what you need to do to reach them can vary with what type of diabetes you have.

For example, if you have gestational diabetes (diabetes that starts during pregnancy), your doctor may have you eat far fewer carbohydrates than the Food Guide Pyramid suggests.

But no matter what kind of diabetes you have, you should put off efforts to lose weight and work on gaining only the weight your doctor advises.

Pregnant women need more of some nutrients. So your doctor will probably suggest that you increase your intake of protein, calcium, iron, and folate.

COMPOSING A DIET

Fat

The *Dietary Guidelines for Americans* advise eating no more than 30% of your calories as fat. Each gram of fat contains 9 calories, so on a 1,200-

calorie-a-day plan to lose weight, 40 grams of fat would be 30% of calories. On a 1,500-calorie meal plan, 50 grams of fat a day would be 30% of calories.

A person who ate a lot of fast food could hit 50 grams pretty fast. That's about the fat in a fast-food hamburger and fries! But what if you eat mostly grains, fruits, and vegetables, as the Food Guide Pyramid suggests, and choose low-fat dairy products and meats? Then staying below 50 grams can be easy. One serving of roasted skinless chicken, broiled round steak, lean ham, steamed or baked fish, or canned tuna has less than 9 grams of fat. An egg has only 2.8 grams of fat.

Also, the guidelines say saturated fat should be less than 10% of your calories. (Saturated fats are found mostly in animal products.)

You don't have to eat this much fat. You can safely eat much less, if you prefer or if your health warrants. (If you have high cholesterol or heart disease, for example, your doctor may suggest limiting saturated fat or total fat even more.) Because fat is naturally present in most foods, even fruits and vegetables, it's hard to eat too little.

If you follow the guidelines for keeping saturated fat low, you will also keep your cholesterol intake low. The foods that are the biggest sources of cholesterol—egg yolks, meats (especially liver and other organ meats), and regular milk products—tend to be high in saturated fat. (When buying packaged foods, always check both fat content and cholesterol, just in case they're not in sync.) It's good to keep your cholesterol intake below 300 milligrams per day. This is the amount in about 3 ounces of cooked beef liver or 1 1/2 eggs.

Protein and Carbohydrate

ADA suggests that people with diabetes get 10% to 20% of their calories from protein. One exception is people with diabetic kidney disease. Often, a diet lower in protein is suggested for them.

Most Americans take in the suggested amount of protein without thinking about it.

In the future, after more research, scientists may be able to pinpoint precisely the best levels of protein, fat, and carbohydrate in the weight-loss diet. But for now, we recommend as the most healthful diet one that contains:

- 30% or fewer calories from fats

- 10% to 20% of calories from proteins

- The rest—perhaps 50% to 70% of calories—from carbohydrates

For a person on a 1,500-calorie diet, this plan means no more than 50 grams of fat (about equal to that in 3 1/2 tablespoons of olive oil) and only 150 to 300 calories from protein (equal to the protein found in 4 1/2 to 9 ounces of steak) each day.

YOUR DIABETES MEAL PLAN

You are already better off than other people in starting healthful eating habits. You've probably already worked with a dietitian on a diabetes-controlling meal plan that's practical for your life. If not, why not make an appointment? Your insurance may cover the cost because dietary advice is part of your medical treatment. (See the box "Talking About Dietitians.")

When you meet with your dietitian, you'll work out a goal for how many calories and what kinds of foods to eat each day. You'll also choose a way to keep track of what you eat. Many people with diabetes count "Exchanges." This system is much like counting the number of servings you're eating from each block of the Food Guide Pyramid. But there are other systems as well.

One popular system is called carbohydrate counting. When blood glucose levels rise after eating, most of that rise is due to the carbohydrates in the meal. In carbohydrate counting, people who take insulin or diabetes pills eat the same amount of carbohydrates each day, spaced the same way through the day. Because, for example, every breakfast contains the same amount of carbohydrate, the rise in glucose afterward should be the same, and the morning insulin or pill dose can be tailored precisely. Later, as people on insulin gain skill in carbohydrate counting, they learn how to adjust their insulin dose when they plan to eat more carbohydrate or less carbohydrate than usual.

Carbohydrate counting is flexible and simple. There's only one nutrient to count, rather than several kinds of Exchanges. But you still

TALKING ABOUT DIETITIANS

What is a dietitian?

A dietitian is a person who has been trained in nutrition. Dietitians who have passed a national test can put RD (registered dietitian) after their names.

Why should I see a dietitian?

A dietitian can help you put together a meal plan that works well for your diabetes and fits the rest of your life as well. For example, if you work odd hours or must travel a lot, your dietitian can help you put together a plan that takes these problems into account and still helps you control your glucose levels and lose weight.

What if I already have a meal plan?

Lives change. Science progresses. People forget. These are three reasons why seeing a dietitian every so often is a good idea. You can refresh your memory and update your meal plan to fit with your current life and the current scientific knowledge about a good diet.

The American Diabetes Association advises seeing a dietitian (or otherwise talking to a professional about your diet) every 6 to 12 months.

Gee, that sounds costly. I worry that my insurance company won't cover my visit.

Some people do have a problem with coverage. But things are getting better.

Many states require insurance companies to cover the cost of diabetes education, and most of the other states are considering similar laws. In addition, Congress has passed a bill to reform Medicare so that it, too, will cover diabetes education.

TALKING ABOUT DIETITIANS *Continued*

If you live in a state with diabetes legislation, it doesn't matter what insurance company you have. It may be required to cover at least some of your dietitian's fee. If you don't live in one of those states, your insurance company may still help cover your visit.

In either case, talk to your insurance company before you see the dietitian. Doing so is very important! Your insurance may pay for your visit only if you go through certain steps first. For example, you may need to get a letter from your doctor and send it to the insurance company. For best results, follow the insurance company's rules to the letter. If you're turned down, appeal.

How do I go about finding a dietitian?

The place to start is with your doctor. He or she should be able to tell you which dietitians in town know a lot about diabetes diets. Some diabetes doctors even have a dietitian on their staff.

If your doctor can't help you, call The American Dietetic Association. (See the RESOURCES section before the index of this book to find out how to contact them.) This association can refer you to registered dietitians in your area.

need to keep an eye on your entire diet. If you pay attention only to carbohydrates, it's easy to eat too much fat and protein and gain weight.

Whatever you do, refuse to accept a preprinted sheet with a one-size-fits-all meal plan. There is no "diabetes diet" that works for everyone with diabetes. ADA stresses that meal plans must be tailored to the people they are for. That means your meal plan must take into account your work schedule, your family duties, what type of diabetes you have, the foods you like and dislike, how often you travel, other health problems you might have, your religion, your ethnic background, and even your income and expenses.

The Skinny on Chapter

7

▶ A good diet is a good diet, whether you are overweight or have diabetes or not.

▶ A reduced-calorie diet is the only way to lose weight.

▶ The Food Guide Pyramid illustrates a healthful diet.

▶ Plant foods should make up most of the diet. Each day, people should eat 6 to 11 servings of grains, 3 to 5 servings of vegetables, and 2 to 4 servings of fruits.

▶ People should also eat 2 to 3 servings of dairy products and 2 to 3 servings of meat, eggs, or beans.

▶ The larger serving numbers are for large or very active people. The smaller serving numbers are suitable for smaller or inactive people or people who are trying to lose weight.

▶ Highly refined foods, such as sugar and oils, should make up only a small part of the diet.

▶ Most scientists believe a diet that derives less than 30% of its calories from fat, and less than 10% of its calories from saturated fat, is best for most people.

▶ Protein should contribute 10% to 20% of the calories for people with healthy kidneys. People with kidney disease should limit their protein.

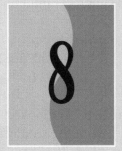

Diets come and go, but one thing doesn't change: Cutting calories is the best way to lose weight.

Cutting Fat and Calories

You are what you eat, according to an old saying. Yet bison become muscular on grassy fare, while many birds stay lean despite feasting on fat-laden seeds or insects. What about humans? Does what you eat matter? Will cutting back on fat in your diet lead to less fat on your body?

The foods you choose do matter in your weight-loss effort. In this chapter, you will learn about the roles of carbohydrates, fats, and proteins in losing weight and controlling glucose. And you'll get some tips on shifting the balance of these nutrients in your diet to a more healthful mix.

CUTTING CALORIES AND WEIGHT LOSS

Losing weight boils down to using more energy than you take in.

This rule of thumb sounds stupidly simple. But putting it into practice is not. For example, it might seem that eating fewer calories or being more active would be two equally useful ways of burning more calories than you eat. In fact, as you will learn in later chapters, exercise helps to improve fitness and to keep pounds off. But it doesn't help much at taking them off in the first place. Only cutting calories does that well. Later in this chapter and again in Chapters 9 and 10, you'll get some tips for cutting calories and adapting the Food Guide Pyramid to your own life.

If you've tried to lose weight before, you may doubt whether cutting calories really works. Research suggests that it does work—but that it's not the complete answer. (See the box "Spotlight on Research: Clinical Trials of Reduced-Calorie Diets.")

Weight Loss in People With Diabetes. Some researchers have looked specifically at whether calorie cutting helps people with diabetes. A study in *Diabetes Care* in 1996 reviewed 89 studies, most published since 1980, containing a total of 1,800 people with diabetes. The review looked not only at how well calorie cutting worked, but also at how it compared with weight-loss drugs, surgery, exercise, and behavioral treatments, alone or in various combinations.

When data from many studies were combined and reanalyzed, the results showed that surgery (which will be discussed in Chapter 16) took off the most pounds. The next most effective treatment was calorie cutting by itself. It took off an average of 20 pounds. Exercise alone took off the fewest pounds—about 3.4 pounds on average. Most of the weight-loss strategies worked better for people younger than 55 than for older people.

Calorie cutting by itself was also best at improving other health measures. It caused glycated hemoglobin (a measure of long-term glucose levels) to drop. Blood pressure, triglycerides (a kind of blood fat), and total cholesterol levels also dropped. One caution about these results: These conclusions depend on the quality of the original studies, and many of these studies did not report changes in measures such as blood pressure. Also, most of the reduced-calorie diets reviewed were very-low-calorie diets. And few studies followed people longer than 6 months after the program ended.

The most important results of this review are:

- People with diabetes can lose weight by cutting calories, just as other people can.

- Eating a low-calorie diet may work better than exercise alone or weight-loss drugs alone in taking off pounds and improving glucose control, blood pressure, and other weight-related health problems.

SPOTLIGHT ON RESEARCH
Clinical Trials of Reduced-Calorie Diets

A 1993 article in *Annals of Internal Medicine* reviewed 65 studies between 1974 and 1990 that combined cutting calories with "behavioral modification." (Behavioral modification means teaching people techniques to help them stick to their weight-loss plan. For example, they might learn to keep a written record of what they eat and when they exercise.) In general, in the 65 studies, women ate a diet of 1,200 calories per day, and men, 1,500 calories per day.

This review found that over the years, the rate of weight loss in studies stayed almost the same: roughly 1 pound per week. The short-term success rate remained the same, too. About half the people managed to lose 20 pounds in 20 weeks.

But there were some differences between the earlier studies (1974 to 1978) and the more recent ones (1984 to 1990). First, the more recent studies lasted longer. As a result, the total weight loss in them was larger. But it became clear in the longest studies that people gradually stopped losing weight.

Second, the studies of 1984 to 1990 tended to follow people longer after they left the weight-loss program. Such studies revealed that in the year after the weight-loss program, people tended to regain about a third of their lost weight. And after that first year, people still tended to keep regaining. After 5 years, most people had returned to their starting weight.

This review suggests that:

- People can lose weight by cutting calories.

- People don't continue losing weight forever, even if they keep up their weight-loss efforts.

- Lost weight often comes back.

This review makes it clear that a reduced-calorie eating plan really does help people lose weight. The next big question is, does it matter what kind of calories—protein, carbohydrates, or fat—you cut?

DOES THE SOURCE OF CALORIES MATTER?

You may not think you know much about "macronutrients," but in fact, your body is a whiz. It quickly sorts what you eat into proteins, fats, and carbohydrates. Each kind of nutrient has a different job, so the body handles each differently.

- Carbohydrates meet day-to-day energy needs. The body converts them into glucose. Some glucose goes to the cells to fuel their activities. Some glucose is stored for a short time in the liver and in muscles until you need it. Foods high in carbohydrates are usually plant foods: vegetables, fruits, beans, grains, and sugar.

- Fats, in contrast, serve a variety of short-term and long-term needs. The body uses some fat energy in everyday living. It stores other fat. Stored fat insulates the body, cushions vital organs, and provides energy in emergencies. Foods high in fat are usually animal foods: meats, dairy products, eggs, and oils.

- Proteins form the structure of the body. The body uses protein from the diet to build tissue. The body can also use protein for fuel when intake of carbohydrates and fats is low. Foods high in protein include meats, dairy products, eggs, beans, and grains.

Low-Fat Diets May Be Best for Losing Weight

Here are five reasons why, in theory, you'll likely lose more weight and keep more off if you cut the amount of fat you eat than if you cut back on carbohydrates or proteins.

- The body tries to use carbohydrates and proteins right away. To avoid storing these nutrients when you eat too many, the body increases its energy use to try to burn them up.

- The amount of fat your body needs for its routine daily chores is quite small. So you can greatly reduce fat in your diet without harm. Not so with protein and carbohydrate. If you were to cut down too much on protein, your body would have trouble repairing itself. If you were to cut down too much on carbohydrates, your body would steal fat and protein from your tissues for energy.

- The body needs carbohydrates and proteins every day. So, some scientists believe, the brain monitors your intake and adjusts your hunger to make sure you're eating the right amounts of these. When you've eaten what you need, the body says "Enough!" by making you feel full. The body might be less fussy about fats. After all, if you eat too much fat, it will just get stored.

- Fat is very high in calories. Each gram has 9 calories, vs. 4 calories per gram in carbohydrates and proteins. It takes very little time to devour a lot of calories when you eat a high-fat food. Chapter 9 will show you how to take advantage of this difference to cut calories while staving off hunger.

- Fat acts as a flavor carrier. It also adds texture and moisture. As a result, high-fat foods often taste very good and feel good in the mouth. And of course, the better something tastes, the easier it is to eat a lot of it. (Don't worry that cutting fat from your diet will make it bland and tasteless! Later in this book, you'll learn many low-calorie tricks for boosting flavor in foods.)

Sugar and Fat Substitutes

Many products nowadays contain fat or sugar substitutes, and the number of such products keeps growing. So researchers have been studying whether they are worth using and whether they are good or bad for you.

Sugar Substitutes. Saccharin, aspartame, and acesulfame K are three artificial sweeteners available for use in the United States. Even though sugar is no longer a forbidden food for people with diabetes, you do need to take account of it in your meal plan. So there may still be a place for artificial sweeteners in your diet. They have no calories. And because they are free foods, they don't use up any Exchanges, either.

Fat Substitutes. There are many fat substitutes, including carrageenan, polydextrose, guar gum, and whey protein concentrates. Most fat substitutes are based on food starches, plant gums and gels, modified egg white, or other carbohydrates or proteins. You might find them in frozen desserts; salad dressings; lunch meats; baked goods such as breads, cookies, and crackers; chewing gum; reduced-fat dairy products such as yogurt and sour cream; soups; sauces; candy—in fact, in almost any packaged food.

SHORT-TERM "DIETS" BEGET SHORT-TERM WEIGHT LOSS

"Fat people know the calories in everything, don't you know?" says Susan Lapin.

Her diets always took weight off in a safe, sensible manner. "I'd take sweets out of my diet," she says. "It wasn't the 'thing' at the time [the early 1960s], but I drank skim milk. I would have a modest lunch—you know, a sandwich, a glass of milk, and a piece of fruit—and a normal dinner without dessert."

Exercise also helped her diets. "When I exercise, I do much better at losing weight," she says. "I would walk a mile briskly because I'd be walking to the bus stop. And my job required me to move around rather briskly, too. And I would sometimes ride my bike to work when I was working at the university here after I got married."

Still, Lapin always gained the weight back eventually. It was hard to stick to her good habits when she was depressed or craved chocolate. And gastritis (irritation of the stomach lining) made her feel hungry all the time. When she reached 346 pounds, she joined a university-based weight-loss program. The doctors encouraged her to eat a reduced-calorie, low-fat diet and become more active, and they put her on weight-loss drugs. The drugs allowed her to control her cravings and lose 75 pounds.

A new type of fat substitute actually is a fat that is altered in structure. Olestra is the most famous of these new fats. These fat substitutes have molecules so big that the body can't digest them. So they just pass through the body and come out in the stool. No energy is absorbed from them. They may cause stomachaches and diarrhea if eaten in more than small amounts.

Safety. The American Diabetes Association believes that approved sugar and fat substitutes are safe. They have survived a rigorous and thorough Food and Drug Administration approval process.

Do Substitutes Help in a Reduced-Calorie Diet? The idea that fat and sugar substitutes help people lose weight assumes that people don't eat more to make up the missing calories. This assumption does not seem to be true.

Scientists have done the most research on sugar substitutes. They have found that people who eat artificially sweetened foods tend to eat more carbohydrates later. So they end up taking in just as many calories. For example, a person might drink sugar-free soft drinks all day and then eat chocolate cake for dessert at night.

What about fat? Only a few studies have looked at whether people who ate fat substitutes took in fewer calories. These studies showed that people who ate fat substitutes later ate more carbohydrates and proteins. So in these studies, the subjects did make up the calories, just not with fat. For instance, a person might eat fat-free cookies, but eat twice as many.

Scientists who reviewed the research on fat substitutes for the American Diabetes Association warned that fat substitutes may affect diabetes control in at least two ways. First, if people really do eat more carbohydrates to make up for the lost fat calories, then they need to take those carbohydrates into account in their meal plan or in their insulin dose. Second, because some fat substitutes are made from carbohydrates, they might raise glucose levels.

Sugar-Free but Not Calorie-Free

There's another kind of sugar substitute. They're called sugar alcohols or polyols. You can usually recognize sugar alcohols because their names end in "ol." Three popular sugar alcohols are sorbitol, mannitol, and xylitol.

Sugar alcohols sometimes appear in products advertised as suitable for people with diabetes. So you may be surprised to find out that they contain calories—about 1 1/2 to 3 calories per gram (vs. 4 calories for sugar). Like sugar, but unlike calorie-free sugar substitutes, sugar alcohols raise blood glucose levels. This rise may be slower and lower with sugar alcohols than with sugar.

Sugar alcohols can upset your intestines or cause diarrhea. For example, sucking on sugarless hard candies all day for a sore throat might be enough to give some adults diarrhea.

KINDS OF FAT

There are three main kinds of fat: saturated, polyunsaturated, and monounsaturated. All three kinds have the same number of calories per gram. So for weight loss, cutting back on all three is equally important.

Not so for good heart health. Monounsaturated fats are the best for you. They lower your cholesterol level. So you should aim to get most of your fat calories from them. The foods that are high in monounsaturated fats are olives, olive oil, and canola oil.

Saturated fats are the worst for your heart. They raise your cholesterol level and put your heart at risk. So you should get as few calories from them as possible. Saturated fat is found mostly in animal foods: meat, egg yolks, whole milk, and whole-milk products such as cheese and butter. Saturated fats also occur in the oils of some tropical plants, such as coconut oil and palm oil.

Polyunsaturated fats fall between saturated and monounsaturated fats in effects on heart health. Like monounsaturated fats, polyunsaturated fats lower cholesterol levels. Most plant fats are polyunsaturated fats. These include safflower oil, sunflower seeds and oil, soybean oil, and corn oil. Peanut oil contains both monounsaturated and polyunsaturated fats.

There's one other fat you should know about: trans fat. It occurs naturally in small amounts in foods that come from cattle and sheep (such as milk and lamb). But most trans fat in the diet comes from artificial sources. It is made by chemically altering liquid polyunsaturated fat to make it hard like saturated fat. This process not only gives the food a more pleasant texture, but also makes it last longer. Margarines and shortenings that are solid at room temperature are two examples of foods with trans fats.

Scientists debate the health effects of trans fats. A task force convened by the American Society for Clinical Nutrition and the American Institute of Nutrition concluded in 1996 that trans fats increase total and "bad" cholesterol levels, but less than saturated fats do. Trans fats may also lower levels of "good" cholesterol. The American Heart Association suggests that people limit trans fats and choose soft margarines rather than stick margarines or butter.

Here are two ways to shift your diet away from saturated fats:

- Base your meals on the Food Guide Pyramid. Doing so can help you eat fewer meats (which tend to be high in saturated fats) and more plant foods (which are low in saturated fats and often in total fats as well).

- Cook with canola oil or olive oil when possible. If you use store-bought salad dressings, margarine, or mayonnaise, look for ones made with canola or olive oil.

WAYS TO CUT FAT FROM YOUR DIET

The fat we eat is often hidden. No greasy shine or slick consistency gives away that apples, corn, and kidney beans all contain a bit of fat. (Of course, that bit is pretty small. Corn on the cob has only 1 gram of fat—far less than the nearly 4 grams of fat in the teaspoon of butter you put on the ear.)

If the only hidden fat was the tiny amount found in nearly every food, including fruits and vegetables, we wouldn't have to worry. But fat has many ways of sneaking into our food without our paying attention. Every time you sauté onions in 1/4 cup of oil, you are adding 56 grams of fat to the dish. Every time you don't skin a chicken breast, you're passing up the chance to remove 4 grams of fat. Here are some ways to reduce the amount of fat, both hidden and visible, that you eat. Chapters 9 and 10 will give you many other ideas.

The Right Equipment

The right tools make any task, including eating less fat, easier.

- Invest in some low-fat cookbooks. Adapting high-fat recipes is tricky and often yields ho-hum results. If a low-fat cookbook's author is a skilled cook, the recipes may taste better than what you could devise on your own.

- A pressure cooker with a self-regulating valve produces flavorful meals with little or no fat. It also lets you cook beans and grains quickly.

- Nonstick pans let you sauté with little or no fat.

- A microwave reheats grains without putting a hard crust on the pot. It is also great for baking potatoes and apples.

- A steaming basket lets you easily cook vegetables, chicken, and fish with no fat.

Shopping

Refraining from high-fat foods is easier if you leave them at the store instead of buying them. To help you do that:

- Plan your menus and write your grocery list after eating, when you are not hungry.

- Shop after eating so that hunger doesn't tempt you to buy extra treats.

- For snacks, try out low-fat and nonfat treats such as pretzels, popcorn (check for low-fat kinds), reduced-fat crackers and chips, graham crackers, sorbet, nonfat frozen yogurt, and nonfat yogurt.

- Read the labels. Competing brands of the same product may vary greatly in fat content. Store-bought spaghetti sauces, for example, vary from 0 to 8 grams of fat per serving.

- Choose the leanest cuts of meat. These come from the hindquarters. All cuts of turkey, chicken, fish, and game animals are relatively low in fat. Even so, white meat of poultry has about half the fat of dark meat. The box "Eight Tips for Choosing Lean Meats" gives more hints for shopping for meats.

- For casseroles, soups, and other medley foods, buy less meat and more vegetables than the recipe calls for.

EIGHT TIPS FOR CHOOSING LEAN MEATS

Americans love meat. Although they make up only 2% of the world's population, Americans eat a third of the meat.

If you, too, love meat, you're probably confused about how to make it part of a healthful, low-calorie diet. Here are eight rules of thumb—and some exceptions—to help you make leaner choices when shopping.

1. Choose mystery meats and other highly processed meats only rarely. Hot dogs, salami, bologna, bacon, and sausages and wursts are high in fat and salt.

Exception #1: Some fake hamburgers and hot dogs contain little or no fat because they're made from soybeans or other vegetables. But when buying fake meats, always read the label. Some have quite a bit of fat and many calories.

Exception #2: A few of the "light" hot dogs, turkey burgers, turkey franks, and turkey lunch meats are much lower in fat than traditional versions. Compare calorie counts and fat grams to find the ones that live up to their light billing. Look for less than 5 grams of fat per serving.

2. Choose cuts from the hindquarters of mammals. These include round and loin cuts of beef, extra-lean (85%) ground beef, loin and leg cuts of pork, lean ham, Canadian bacon, and loin and leg cuts of lamb.

Continued

EIGHT TIPS FOR CHOOSING LEAN MEATS *Continued*

3. When buying graded meat, choose Select grade. In the past, fatty meat was thought the best kind. So the highest grade, Prime, is awarded to the fattiest meat. Select grade is the "worst" (leanest) grade, and Choice meat falls in between.

4. Choose organ meats only rarely. These include liver, tongue, kidney, and sweetbreads. All are high in cholesterol.

5. Choose seafood more often than meat from mammals. Fish and other seafood tend to be lower in fat, particularly saturated fat. Also, the so-called omega fatty acids in fish and other seafood are thought to be good for the heart.

Exception #1: Fish canned in oil is high in calories and fat. For example, most tuna canned in water has only 1 or 2 grams of fat per serving (depending on the brand and type). But tuna canned in oil might have 10 or more grams of fat per serving—doubling the calorie count.

Exception #2: Caviar (fish eggs) is high in fat and cholesterol.

6. Choose poultry more often than meat from mammals. Like fish, poultry tends to be low in fat, especially saturated fat. White meat contains less fat than dark meat.

Exception #1: Eggs are high in fat and cholesterol.

Exception #2: Ducks and geese, as you might guess from their rounded shapes, tend to be fatty.

Exception #3: Poultry skin is high in fat.

7. Choose game meats if you have a safe source. Wild animals (for example, deer, turtle, buffalo, and pheasant) tend to be lower in fat than farm animals.

8. No matter what meat you are choosing, look for as little visible fat as possible. Meats of the same grade or cut can still vary in how much fat they have. By looking them over, you can choose the package with the least extra fat and later cut off whatever fat you can see.

Cooking Methods

Cooking methods have a big effect on the fat content of dishes. Here are some ways to lighten up.

- Sauté with less than a tablespoon of oil. In fact, spritzing your pan lightly with nonstick cooking spray may be enough if you stir the foods often.

- Instead of sautéing onions, garlic, and green peppers, try softening them by cooking them briefly in the microwave.

- Sauté in 1/4 cup of wine or defatted broth instead of butter or oil.

- Bake, steam, grill, broil, poach, or roast, when possible.

- Remove fat and skin from meats.

- Thicken a soup by puréeing some of it rather than by adding cream or sour cream.

- Choose sauces thickened with cornstarch or arrowroot instead of with eggs, cream, or cheese.

- Grate or finely chop high-fat garnishes (such as olives, cheese, nuts, or chocolate) so that you can use less, yet each bite will still contain some of the flavor.

- Cook chicken or fish en papillote (that is, wrapped and sealed in cooking parchment or foil). This fast and easy technique preserves all the moisture, so these meats come out tender and juicy. The steam also infuses the meat with flavor if you add herbs, ginger slices, or leek strips to the packets.

- Marinate without oil. Marinades can be based on lemon juice, lime juice, wine, broth, nonfat yogurt, fat-free salad dressing, or tomato juice.

- If you use packaged foods, don't feel bound to the directions. For example, if the package calls for 1/2 cup of whole milk, try skim milk instead. If it calls for a tablespoon of butter, try 1 or 2 teaspoons instead.

Substitutes

You'll need to experiment to learn which low-fat and nonfat ingredients you like. Many people find a gulf between the tastes of low-fat foods and their nonfat counterparts. If you do, too, you may prefer to use low-fat substitutes.

Table 8-1 lists substitutions you can try in recipes. Table 8-2 lists other kinds of substitutes. To prevent unpleasant surprises, try out a substitute before using it in a dish for company!

Cutting a lot of fat does not always mean you are cutting a lot of calories. Often, low-fat recipes call for more sugar or fruit than usual to make up for the loss of fat flavor, adding calories.

CUTTING CALORIES WHEN YOU HAVE DIABETES

Because you have diabetes, your weight-loss eating plan also needs to keep your glucose levels under control. These two goals—weight loss and diabetes control—mesh together well. In fact, a reduced-calorie diet has

TABLE 8-1

Low-Fat Substitutes for Recipes

WHEN A RECIPE CALLS FOR:	TRY INSTEAD:
An egg	■ Two egg whites, or ■ 1/4 cup of egg substitute
Whole milk	■ Skim milk
Sour cream	■ Low-fat or nonfat sour cream, or ■ Low-fat or nonfat yogurt, or ■ Two parts low-fat cottage cheese puréed with one part buttermilk
Light cream	■ Whole milk, or ■ Nonfat buttermilk

TABLE 8-1 *Continued*

WHEN A RECIPE CALLS FOR:	TRY INSTEAD:
Whipping (heavy) cream	■ Evaporated skim milk
Cottage cheese	■ Low-fat or nonfat cottage cheese
Cheese	■ A small amount of a very sharp cheese, or ■ Low-fat or nonfat cheese
Cream cheese	■ Nonfat cream cheese, or ■ Neufchâtel cheese
Mayonnaise	■ Low-fat or nonfat mayonnaise
Shortening-based pie crust (for sweet pies)	■ Crumb crust, or ■ Meringue crust (if the pie will not be cooked after filling)
Eggs and oil in baked goods	■ An equal amount of nonfat yogurt
Butter or oil in sweet baked goods	■ Half as much applesauce, or ■ Half as much of a fruit-based butter and oil replacement
Tuna in oil	■ Tuna in water
Hamburger	■ Ground turkey, or ■ Cooked beans or soaked bulgur in place of part of the meat
Veal cutlets	■ Turkey cutlets
Tofu	■ Low-fat tofu
Nuts (in a bread)	■ Raisins or other dried fruit, or ■ A smaller amount of toasted nuts
Nuts (in a salad)	■ Water chestnuts, cut into small chunks
Chocolate (in baking)	■ Cocoa powder (for each ounce of chocolate, use 3 Tbs. of cocoa; you may also need to add 1 tsp. of oil)

TABLE 8-2

Other Low-Fat Substitutes

WHEN YOU WOULD USE:	TRY INSTEAD:
Cream cheese (as a topping)	■ Nonfat cream cheese, or ■ Neufchâtel cheese
Mayonnaise (as a topping)	■ Low-fat or nonfat mayonnaise
Butter (as a bread topping)	■ Puréed fruit spreads, or ■ Nonfat cream cheese, or ■ Neufchâtel cheese, or ■ Roasted, mashed garlic
Butter (as a vegetable topping)	■ Low-fat or nonfat sour cream, or ■ Low-fat cottage cheese, or ■ Lemon juice and garlic, or ■ Fresh salsa
Nondairy coffee whitener	■ Evaporated skim milk
Ice cream	■ Sorbet

great effects on diabetes even when it fails as a strategy for major weight loss:

- Your glucose control is likely to improve, sometimes within a few days.

- You and your doctor may be able to lower your dose of diabetes pills or insulin or even stop them altogether.

- Surprisingly, your glucose control may improve even if you don't lose a lot of weight. That is, cutting calories helps you two ways. It may lower your weight, which then lowers your glucose level. And it may improve your glucose level directly.

JOINING A WEIGHT-LOSS PROGRAM

Joining some kind of weight-loss group or program appeals to many people. About 13% of women and 5% of men sign up for an organized weight-loss program when they want to lose weight.

Kinds of Programs

Weight-loss programs fall into three categories. They vary in type of supervision, method of weight loss, and cost.

Support Groups. In support groups, you meet with other people who are trying to lose weight. You talk about your problems and successes and encourage each other's efforts. They offer no prescribed eating or exercise program and no counseling. Groups may meet every week. Although members run the group, outside speakers may be invited. These programs typically cost very little (less than $20 per year). These are the cheapest programs, but they don't provide any professional advice. Examples of support groups are Overeaters Anonymous and Take Off Pounds Sensibly.

Nonclinical Programs. In nonclinical programs, counselors guide you in eating a reduced-calorie diet and learning to change your behavior. The programs focus on learning to eat less. Some also encourage exercise. In some of these, you may need to buy your food from the program. Costs vary widely, depending on how long you stay in the program (some charge a weekly fee), whether you buy the program's line of foods, and whether you buy other items such as vitamins or motivational tapes and videos. These programs also vary in their philosophies and the soundness of their advice. To join some of these programs, people with diabetes must have written permission from their doctor. Examples of nonclinical programs are Diet Center, Jenny Craig, Nutri/System, and Weight Watchers.

Clinical Programs. These programs are run by health care professionals (usually doctors, nurses, dietitians, and/or psychologists). They may consist of supervised diets of no more than 800 calories a day for 3 to 4 months. These may include liquid diets that remove the need to count calories or make food choices. (See Chapter 14 for an in-depth look at very-low-calorie diets.) Some of these programs offer traditional low-calorie diet plans as well. Others may offer drug treatment to people who are very overweight. (See Chapter 15 for a closer look at weight-loss drugs.) Some programs also provide weekly group meetings and one-on-one counseling.

Very-low-calorie diet programs are the most costly of the weight-loss programs and often cost $2,000 or more—although your insurance may cover some of the fee. Some require people with type 1 diabetes to get a letter of permission from their doctor; some exclude people with type 1 altogether. Very-low-calorie diets and weight-loss drugs must be supervised by a reputable doctor. Examples of clinical programs are Health Management Resources, Medifast, New Direction, and Optifast.

Choosing a Nonclinical Weight-Loss Program

Several years ago, the National Institutes of Health and the Food and Drug Administration tried to collect information about how well different weight-loss programs work. To the dismay of scientists and overweight people alike, many companies did not respond, and the data sent were often skimpy. The government scientists could not draw any conclusions about the success rates of nonclinical programs.

So how do you go about choosing a program? Start first with your doctor. He or she may know the reputations of the programs in your area and can steer you away from bad ones. Also, your doctor or clinic may offer a program.

Next, talk to people from each nonclinical program you are thinking about. Ask many questions. You'll want to find out not only general information about the program, but also how well suited it is for people with diabetes. Here are some sample questions to ask:

- What is the cost of the program?

- What does that fee cover? What is extra?

- What percentage of people drop out?

- How much weight do people keep off after 1 year? After 5 years? What is the source of those numbers?

- Who runs your program?

- Are any nurses, doctors, dietitians, or psychologists part of the program? What preparation and training have they had?

- Does your program include behavioral modification? How about exercise or nutrition advice?

- How many pounds a week do you encourage people to lose? (More than 1 or 2 pounds a week may be too much.)

- What is the scientific basis for your diet? Does it reflect the *Dietary Guidelines for Americans*?

- How suitable is your plan for people with diabetes?

- Do I buy my meals from you or make my own?

- Are any foods forbidden? Why?

- What risks does your program have?

- How long does the program last?

- Is there a maintenance program to join after I lose weight?

 The
Skinny on
Chapter

 8

▶ Studies show that people who cut calories do lose weight.

▶ Weight loss usually tapers off after awhile. Then, if people do not take steps to keep weight off, lost weight often comes back.

▶ For most people, maintaining weight loss needs at least as much attention as losing weight in the first place.

▶ Cutting calories works just as well for people with diabetes as it does for other people.

▶ The easiest way to cut calories for weight loss may be to cut mostly fat calories, but be sure you don't add in more carbohydrates or proteins.

▶ Cutting fat calories without cutting total calories will lead to little or no weight loss.

▶ There are three types of weight-loss programs: support groups, nonclinical programs, and clinical programs. They vary in type of supervision, method of weight loss, and cost.

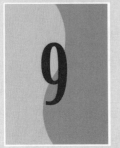

9

Your tastes in food are not set in stone. You and your family can learn to enjoy a wide variety of healthful foods.

The American Way of Eating

Would you eat coagulated animal body secretions? What if they contained mold colonies? Would you add spoiled wine or funguses to your recipe?

You probably have. And you probably thought they were yummy. Most people like cheese and yogurt (coagulated milk). Gorgonzola cheese, stinky as it is, is beloved by many, despite containing mold. And many recipes call for vinegar (spoiled wine) or mushrooms (funguses).

Some food preferences are inborn. But in general, humans can learn to enjoy all sorts of things, from moldy cheeses to overly fermented wine. This chapter will help you think about what you eat and why. To lose weight and keep it off, you must adopt healthful eating habits and keep them forever. If you don't like healthful foods, this plan might sound like a recipe for torture. But in fact, people can learn to like a healthful diet. This chapter will show you how.

HOW DOES YOUR DIET STACK UP?

Here's a test for you. Don't get nervous! There's no time limit and no grade. This test will just give you some data on your own eating habits and beliefs to compare with the rest of America—and with what scientists believe is the most healthful diet.

1. From which of the five food groups—Meat and Beans, Milk, Grain Products, Vegetable, or Fruit—do you eat the most foods?

———————————————————————————————

2. How many servings of fruit do you eat each day?

———————————————————————————————

3. Do you get all the calcium you need? What foods do you get it from?

———————————————————————————————

4. How many servings of vegetables do you eat each day?

———————————————————————————————

5. Are you eating the right amount of protein? From what foods do you get most of your protein?

———————————————————————————————

6. How varied is your diet? Do you eat a wide variety of foods or mostly the same foods over and over?

———————————————————————————————

7. Do you limit how much fat and cholesterol you eat?

———————————————————————————————

8. How much alcohol do you drink?

———————————————————————————————

9. How much salt do you eat?

———————————————————————————————

10. How much sugar do you eat?

———————————————————————————————

How Does Your Diet Compare With What's Best?

If the quiz questions sounded familiar, it's not surprising. Most of the questions are based on the diet advice of the *Dietary Guidelines for Americans,* which was the subject of Chapter 7. There, you learned the guidelines themselves and some of the reasons for them. Now, it's time to see how your diet compares with the one suggested by experts.

Question 1: The Five Food Groups. The *Dietary Guidelines for Americans* suggest that foods from the Grain Products Group make up the bulk of the diet (in both senses of the word!). They advise that Americans eat 6 to 11 servings of bread, cereal, rice, and pasta each day.

Questions 2 and 4: Fruits and Vegetables. The *Dietary Guidelines for Americans* suggest that fruits and vegetables be plentiful in the diet. They advise three to five servings of vegetables and two to four servings of fruits each day.

Question 3: Calcium. The *Dietary Guidelines for Americans* suggest that people eat two to three servings each day of milk, yogurt, and cheese, the most calcium-rich foods. A National Institutes of Health (NIH) Consensus Conference in 1994 gave this advice:

- Adults younger than 24 should take in 1,200 to 1,500 milligrams of calcium each day.

- Women who are pregnant or breastfeeding should also take in 1,200 to 1,500 milligrams per day.

- Women who have passed menopause and are not taking estrogen should take in 1,500 milligrams per day.

- Everyone over 65 should take in at least 1,500 milligrams a day.

- Other women and all men between 24 and 65 should take in at least 1,000 milligrams per day.

For most people, the NIH advice translates into 3 to 5 servings of calcium-rich foods a day (a little higher than the *Dietary Guidelines for*

Americans suggest). Eight ounces of skim milk contains 302 milligrams of calcium. A cup of nonfat yogurt can have more than 400. Many cheeses have between 150 and 200 milligrams per ounce.

Question 5: Protein. According to the *Dietary Guidelines for Americans,* people need two to three servings from the Meat and Beans Group each day. This high-protein food group includes red meat, poultry, fish, dried beans, eggs, and nuts.

Question 6: Variety. The *Dietary Guidelines for Americans* suggest that people eat a variety of foods. Variety is good because no food has every nutrient you need. Milk is high in protein and low in vitamin C; the opposite is true of orange juice. A 1997 study in the *Journal of the American Dietetic Association* found that eating a variety of foods each day was linked to getting more vitamins and less fat. This tendency may help explain why people who eat foods from several food groups each day are less likely to die from heart disease and cancer.

Question 7: Fat and Cholesterol. The *Dietary Guidelines for Americans* say to choose a diet low in fat and cholesterol. They suggest that people take in less than 30% of their calories from fat and less than 300 milligrams of cholesterol a day.

Question 8: Alcohol. The American Diabetes Association (ADA) guidelines say that some people who use insulin or sulfonylurea drugs can drink alcohol with a meal. People who drink alcohol should do so in moderation. "Moderation" means one drink per day for women and two drinks per day for men. "One drink" means 12 ounces of beer, 5 ounces of wine, or 1 1/2 ounces of 80-proof hard liquor. For people who count Exchanges, one drink equals two Fat Exchanges.

Question 9: Salt. The *Dietary Guidelines for Americans* suggest that salt be enjoyed in moderation. ADA agrees. They suggest that people with diabetes who have high blood pressure should eat less than 2,400 milligrams of sodium each day, and those with high blood pressure and kidney disease eat less than 2,000 milligrams a day.

Question 10: Sugar. The *Dietary Guidelines for Americans* suggest that sugar be enjoyed in moderation. ADA also says that sugar consumed as part of the meal plan does not hurt glucose control. But if people eat sugar, they should take account of it in their meal plan.

WITH A LITTLE HELP FROM HIS FAMILY

When Stephan Windrum got diabetes, he decided to lose weight so that he could live to see his kids and grandkids grow up. His whole family pitched in to help. His wife changed her grocery-buying habits so that she brings home the foods he should have. She also measures his food. His daughter keeps track of how much sugar he eats.

In fact, the whole family is eating better now. "They more or less eat what I can have," Windrum says. "They eat the stuff that's good for me, not just stuff that they want."

The American Diet and You

What if this brief quiz shows that your diet is not up to snuff? What if you thought you were eating a good diet? If so, it's clear from the statistics that you're in sync with most Americans. It's hard to keep up with changes in scientific knowledge.

But it's never too late to change your meals for the better. This chapter will show you how people learn to like and dislike certain foods. Throughout this chapter and Chapter 10, as in Chapters 7 and 8, you'll get tips for cutting calories and fat while enjoying what you eat and avoiding hunger.

WHERE TASTES COME FROM

What foods you like and don't like depend on many factors:

- Your culture and upbringing

- Your age

- Your genes

■ Your sex

■ Your medical conditions

As you can see, some reasons you like what you like are unchangeable, but not all of them. Knowing how tastes form will help you learn to like new foods that may seem strange at first, just as you once may have made an effort to learn to like artichokes or wine or coffee.

Your Genes

Most human groups have adopted settled lifestyles and taken up agriculture in the past 10,000 years. But that is just the blink of an eye compared with the millions of years that humans roamed from place to place, hunting game and gathering wild plants. Our biology has not changed much with a mere 10,000 years of civilization. Today, human tastes still reflect the environments people lived in through most of prehistory.

The taste for salt may be inborn, for example. In the hot tropical regions where most humans lived for so long, it's easy to sweat away a lot of salt quickly. But salt is uncommon in these regions. So the people who survived were those who ate salt when they found it and those who conserved salt well.

Cravings for sweets also seem to be genetic. Even a newborn baby will suck sweet liquids with enthusiasm, but make a face in response to bitter or sour tastes. Because sweet foods are often high in calories, a sweet tooth helped people survive when getting enough energy was a daily challenge.

If you lived in a very poor country, liking salty and high-calorie foods best would help keep you alive. But in the United States, most people have plenty of food. So we no longer need to worry about getting enough energy or about getting enough of some nutrients. These inborn taste preferences are no longer useful in guiding our food choices.

Some inherited tastes differ among people. For example, a certain form of one gene affects how well people can taste bitter substances and how sweet and hot foods taste. The proportion of people with this form varies

FUN FRENCH FRY FACTS

- Nearly one-quarter of the vegetable intake of American children consists of french fries.

- Despite Americans' love for fries, the United States is fifth in the world in potato production. Russia is first.

- Potatoes originated in Central and South America, where they were grown 4,000 years ago.

- It's unknown where french fries were invented. The word "french" means to cut into strips.

- The first American to serve french fries was Thomas Jefferson.

- One small bag of 20 to 25 thin french fries counts as a whopping 2 Carbohydrate Exchanges and 2 Fat Exchanges.

- Fast food restaurants make it easier to eat more than 20 fries. The standard 3-ounce bag of fries has 274 calories and 14 grams of fat. But a super-sized serving can weigh twice that. For example, the super-size fries at one popular chain have 540 calories and 26 grams of fat.

- What if you could get rid of the fat? Then you'd have a nutrition powerhouse. If you removed the fat in those super-size fries, you'd cut 234 calories. But they would still provide 8 grams of protein, 6 grams of fiber, and a third of the daily vitamin C requirement.

- Baked "fries" are easy and tasty. To make, cut potatoes into pieces the size of fries. (Allow about 6 ounces—1 medium potato—per person). Toss potato pieces with olive oil. (Use about 1/2 teaspoon per person.) Place on a baking sheet lightly sprayed with nonstick spray. Sprinkle lightly with paprika and salt, if desired. Bake at 475°F for 25 minutes.

greatly among ethnic groups, but in every group, most people have it and are extra sensitive to bitter tastes. To people with this gene form, the caffeine in a cup of coffee tastes bitter, and chili peppers sear the mouth. Such inborn taste preferences may sway your choice of foods. Some scientists believe that people who are sensitive to bitter tastes may be more likely to dislike cabbage-family vegetables such as brussels sprouts and broccoli, which contain bitter compounds.

Your Age

Foods taste different to people of different ages.

Young children adore very sweet foods. From the time they're born until they start to mature, children have a sweet tooth. But during the teen years, this taste preference wanes.

The senses of taste and smell decline after age 60. Foods may have less flavor or aroma than before, may taste or smell odd, or may become totally tasteless or odorless.

Your Sex

Men and women may differ in which foods they love the best. In a study of obese people, men's favorite foods tended to be meat, fish, and eggs. Women's favorite foods tended to be ice cream, chocolate, cake, cookies, doughnuts, and pies.

Your Health

Many illnesses and drugs can change the way foods taste or smell. For example, some sulfonylurea diabetes pills affect the sense of taste. So do other common drugs, such as some antibiotics and blood pressure drugs. And diabetes itself can change the way foods taste.

Your Family and Cultural Heritage

In general, people like what they're used to eating. For example, humans seem to have an inborn dislike for bitter foods. Newborn babies reject sour and bitter substances. Even so, in many cultures, people learn to like sour or bitter foods. On a typical day, 87% of women and 80% of men in the United States drink bitter beverages (coffee or tea). Similarly, many people learn to tolerate or even love hot peppers by eating them.

Some researchers believe that the "fat tooth" in Western culture is acquired the same way. Children may learn to like high-fat foods by eating lots of them when they're little.

Cultures also have rules about what foods are acceptable or not acceptable. In some religions, pigs are thought unfit for eating. In some parts of India, cows are considered sacred and are not eaten. In the United States, bugs are considered unfit food—even though they are quite nutritious. (See the box "Bug Bites.")

Learning to like what your family eats starts young, perhaps even before you're born. Some of the foods a nursing mother eats flavor her milk. Later, children imitate their parents and their friends in many ways, including eating.

Changing Your Tastes

The scientific research on taste shows that even though some preferences are inborn, learning plays a huge role in what foods you like. So you can take charge of your tastes and change them to fit your new lifestyle.

Salt. To learn to like your food less salty, eat less salt. The amount of salt you like is tied to how much you usually eat. If you lower that amount, the natural flavors of your food will come out. Over time, you will learn to prefer the real flavor of food and not want it buried by salt. Some studies suggest it takes taste buds only 8 to 12 weeks to adjust to a lower salt content.

Fat. How people can learn to prefer a low-fat, low-cholesterol diet is less clear. Because fat holds flavor, foods reduced in fat are often less tasty. Some researchers think eating less fat will change your tastes, but others disagree.

On the other hand, eating a food over and over can increase how much you like it. If you choose to eat more vegetables, fruits, beans, and grain foods, you will come to like them more and more. Then you will have many low-fat foods that you like to choose from.

BUG BITES

Can you separate myths about eating insects from fact?

People don't eat bugs.

False. In fact, most people do. Europeans and North Americans are the exception in their loathing for insects. In most places in the world, locusts, grasshoppers, crickets, ants, termites, and the larvae of moths, beetles, and butterflies are well liked.

Bugs are too dirty to eat.

False. Bugs carry no more diseases than mammals or birds. All foods that come from living creatures can carry funguses, viruses, bacteria, and other things that can make you sick. But proper cooking kills these organisms. Like meat, insects are usually eaten fried or roasted.

Bugs aren't nutritious.

False. Insects have lots of protein, and many are dense with calories, making them a good food when other food supplies are short. In fact, the Bible says that after the Hebrews fled Egypt, they ate manna in the wilderness to survive. According to one theory, manna was an insect excretion.

Bugs can be a good addition to a low-calorie diet.

Not usually. Many insects are high in fat and calories. For example, 3 1/2 ounces of broiled lean ground beef has 17.6 grams of fat and 272 calories. In contrast, 3 1/2 ounces of African termites has 46 grams of fat and 610 calories. Clearly, African termites are not a low-calorie food.

The authors of this book enjoy eating bugs.

False. Knowing that a food prejudice has no basis in fact doesn't make it go away!

Also, you can give more flavor to low-fat foods by choosing the right cooking and flavoring methods. Chapters 8 and 10 list many ways to add zing to low-fat foods.

Widening Your Diet. People seem to differ genetically in how sensitive they are to bitter, sweet, and hot tastes. So preferences for these flavors are harder to deal with. Think about how you react to these tastes in foods and how you can work around them or make them work for you. For example, if you love hot foods, you may find you can relish many vegetables you disliked by dousing them with chilies or chili-based sauces. If you hate bitter foods, you may be able to enjoy them by using long-cooking methods, which sweeten onions and cabbage-family vegetables.

DIETS OF THE FIRST AMERICANS

Science progresses. Modern medicine can cure many diseases. Modern technology protects us from frostbite, sunburn, mosquitoes, and other threats better than ever before.

But in some other fields, what occurs is change, not progress. People can argue for hours about which era or country produced the best art, music, or food.

In some ways, the modern diet doesn't measure up to what our ancestors ate. In the United States, much diabetes research has focused on native peoples. Diabetes, once unknown among American Indians, has exploded among some groups to become a huge health menace. A century ago, no Pima Indians had diabetes. Today, more than half of the Pima over 35 who live in Arizona have type 2 diabetes. And the Pima are not alone. Type 2 diabetes has become rampant among the Sioux, Chippewa, Pueblo, Cherokee, and other Indian tribes, as well as native Hawaiians.

What's going on? Some scientists think they are seeing the "thrifty gene" hypothesis in action. As you may remember from Chapter 1, when food is scarce, people who store energy easily (that is, put on fat easily) are at an advantage. They are more likely to survive famines than people whose bodies burn more energy. Scientists believe that the Pima as a people have a high genetic tendency to store fat and to get type 2 diabetes.

The Pima were lean and healthy when the tribe ate beans, acorns, prickly pear fruits, corn, squash, game, and fish. In this diet, roughly 15% of calories came from fat. But in the late 1800s, non-Indian farmers diverted the Pima's water supply. Unable to farm without water, the Pima were forced to accept government handouts of lard, sugar, and white flour to survive. After World War II, the Pima gave up the rest of their native diet to eat high-fat Western foods. They also adopted a sedentary lifestyle like other Americans. As a result, today, more than 70% of Pima in their 20s have BMIs above 27, and the leading cause of death is diabetic kidney disease. (See the box "Spotlight on Research: So Near and Yet So Far.")

Next to the Pima, the heaviest people in the United States are native Hawaiians. And like the Pima, native Hawaiians have high rates of diabetes. One group has been promoting the idea that native Hawaiians should return to elements of a traditional Hawaiian lifestyle, including eating a traditional low-fat, high-fiber diet. This so-called Waianae diet stresses native Hawaiian plants and plant foods such as taro, poi, breadfruit, and sweet potatoes.

In a small study of this diet reported in the *American Journal of Clinical Nutrition* in 1991, 19 native Hawaiians adopted it for 21 days. All 19 were obese and so were greatly at risk for heart disease. On the diet, they took in only 7% of their calories as fat. (People in Hawaii get 38% of their calories from fat on average.) Everyone was urged to eat until full. Even so, the people averaged 1,000 fewer calories per day. They lost an average of 17 pounds each in the 3 weeks of the study. Their cholesterol levels, glucose levels, and blood pressure dropped.

This study, brief and small as it was, shows how eating bulky foods low in fat lets people eat until full while greatly lowering their calorie intake. The authors credited pride in Hawaiian culture as part of the reason the subjects were able to stick to their food plan.

So there's good news. The message from studies of native diets is that people who are prone to overweight and diabetes should not resign themselves to a life of bad health. These studies show that eating a healthful diet and being active can lead to weight loss even in people who are genetically prone to conserve calories, such as the Pima and native Hawaiians. These diets also provide models for other Americans who are looking to improve their diets.

SPOTLIGHT ON RESEARCH
So Near and Yet So Far

A study published in *Diabetes Care* in 1994 shows clearly the effect of diet on overweight and diabetes among the Pima. Researchers compared the lifestyle of the Pima of Arizona with that of an isolated small group of Pima who live in Mexico. The Mexican Pima have been slower to adopt a Western lifestyle. Their diet, which relies heavily on tortillas, beans, and potatoes, is not very good. It is boring and lacks fruits and vegetables. Even so, it has some advantages over the Western diet of the Arizona Pima. It's high in fiber, low in refined carbohydrates, and low in fat. Also, the Mexican Pima men tend to work strenuous jobs.

If the Pima of Arizona and the Pima of Mexico are genetically close, as researchers suspect, then differences between them in rates of obesity and diabetes are likely due to their lifestyles. The researchers compared 35 Mexican Pima with 350 Arizona Pima. The Mexican Pima were much less likely to have diabetes. Only 6% of men and 11% of women among the Mexican Pima had diabetes, compared with 54% of men and 37% of women among the Arizona Pima. Weights were much lower, too. The Mexican women had an average body mass index (BMI) of 25.1, and the men, 24.8. Among the Arizona Pima, women's BMIs averaged 35.5, and men's BMIs averaged 30.8.

Despite their harsh life and inadequate diet, the Mexican Pima were healthier in some ways than Arizona Pima. This study suggests that because they were very active and ate a somewhat traditional diet low in fat, the Mexican Pima were able to avoid getting fat and getting diabetes.

The Skinny on Chapter

9

- ▶ Listening to what your body tells you is not always a good idea. Your body is programmed to urge you to eat salty, high-calorie foods.
- ▶ People are born liking sweets and disliking bitter foods.
- ▶ Some people genetically are more sensitive to bitter tastes than others.
- ▶ Children like sweeter food than adults do.
- ▶ Older people's taste preferences can change as aging affects how well they can taste and smell.
- ▶ Many diseases and drugs, including diabetes pills, can affect how foods taste or smell.
- ▶ Eating a certain food often leads to liking it. For this reason, people are likely to enjoy the foods their family and other people in their culture eat.
- ▶ Women and men may differ in what foods they like best.
- ▶ In the United States, as native peoples have adopted the Western lifestyle, they have also acquired high rates of obesity and diabetes.

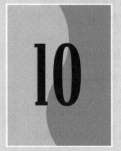

CHAPTER

10

You can still delight in the joys of eating as part of a healthful lifestyle.

Surprise! You Can Eat a Tasty, Filling Diet

E ating is fun. In fact, eating is one of the most fun things you can do. People often reward themselves with a dinner out. Families celebrate birthdays, anniversaries, and holidays by eating a big meal. Courting couples often get to know each other at the dinner table. Even cats can be persuaded to learn a trick if you offer a tasty-enough treat.

Some people hesitate to adopt healthful eating habits because they fear life will no longer be fun. They picture themselves gloomily chomping celery sticks while their friends laugh and feast. Or they worry they will be hungry all the time.

Healthful food **can** be filling and give you joy. Chapters 7 and 8 introduced you to what scientists know about good nutrition and how cutting calories can help you lose weight. But how to translate that knowledge into tasty, hearty breakfasts, lunches, and dinners day after day is not always clear. Earlier chapters gave you some suggestions. This chapter focuses completely on practical hints for changing how you eat. You'll learn how to expand the universe of foods you eat; how to avoid hunger by choosing filling, satisfying foods; and how to avoid the temptation to overdo at social events.

120

EATING SO YOU DON'T FEEL DEPRIVED

Some people get hungry soon after meals when they start eating fewer calories. But constant hunger does not have to go hand in hand with eating healthier. In fact, it can't, if you are to have any hope of keeping up healthful eating habits for the rest of your life! Learning which foods are most satisfying will enable you to choose a filling diet.

What Makes People Feel Full

Some researchers have explored what makes people feel full. Rather than comparing different foods, most have focused on comparing types of nutrients. That is, do protein, carbohydrate, and fat make people feel equally full? Do other qualities of food make them more or less filling? Does a high-fiber diet keep your stomach full longer? One way to explore these questions is to see how long animals or people wait before eating again after eating a certain kind of food. Or scientists can measure the effect of a certain food on how much animals or people eat later. Yet another way is to measure how much is eaten in a day when the diet is high in a particular food type vs. a day when the diet is low in that food.

These three methods share a common assumption: The more filling and satisfying a food is, the longer it takes before hunger strikes, and the fewer the calories people will eat. But some scientists think this assumption is false. They believe that a calorie is a calorie and that people tend to eat the same number of calories, no matter what foods the calories are in. Scientists have a lot to learn about what makes a food filling. Even so, some kinds of foods do seem to make it easier to stick to a reduced-calorie diet.

Foods That Are High in Fiber. Some scientists believe that high-fiber foods make you feel full by keeping food in your stomach longer. Keep in mind that foods that come from animals have no fiber. Fiber comes from plant foods. So cheese, beef, pork, lamb, fish, milk, and eggs provide no fiber. Fruits, vegetables, grains, and beans do. One apple has about 3 grams of fiber, 3/4 cup of cooked oatmeal has 1.6 grams, and 1 cup of cooked kidney beans has 6.4 grams. (See the box "Talking About Fiber" to learn more about the different kinds of fiber and their effects on health.)

TALKING ABOUT FIBER

What is fiber, anyway?

Fiber is sometimes defined as the parts of plants that can't be digested.

If the body doesn't digest fiber, then how can it be good to eat?

Fiber has several good effects:

- By increasing the fiber you eat, you are likely to eat more nutrient-rich foods that are low in fat and calories. This benefit occurs because fiber is found in grains, beans, vegetables, and fruits, especially the less-processed ones.

- Insoluble fiber adds bulk to stools. So it works well to treat or prevent constipation.

- Soluble fiber lowers cholesterol levels.

- Fiber may lower the risk of colon cancer.

Insoluble fiber? Soluble fiber? What's the difference?

In the laboratory, scientists can subject food substances such as fiber to all sorts of treatments. When they put fiber into acid, some dissolves (soluble fiber) and some doesn't (insoluble fiber). Good sources of soluble fiber are oats, beans, brown rice, peas, carrots, and many fruits. A good source of insoluble fiber is wheat bran, which is found in some breakfast cereals and in whole-wheat flour. Because the stomach uses acid to digest food, it's possible that these two types of fiber digest differently in the body just as they do in the lab. In any case, they do have different effects on health.

TALKING ABOUT FIBER *Continued*

How much fiber do I need?

The American Diabetes Association recommends that people with diabetes eat 20 to 35 grams of fiber each day.

How do I make sure I take in enough fiber?

As with most nutrients, eating a diet based on the Food Guide Pyramid is a big step toward getting enough fiber. One easy way to boost fiber intake is by having cereal for breakfast or a snack. Look for cereals with at least 5 grams of fiber per serving.

You don't need to worry about the different kinds of fiber. If you eat a variety of whole grains, fruits, and vegetables, you will take in both soluble and insoluble fiber.

When I tried increasing my fiber before, I got cramps and diarrhea. I don't want to go through that again!

If you are not used to eating foods with fiber, try adding them to your diet slowly. At the same time, increase how much water you drink. These two steps will let your body adjust slowly.

Foods That Are Not Dense in Calories. It would be hard work to eat 500 calories of carrots. That's more than two and a half pounds! But 500 calories of some ice creams is less than a cup and disappears in a flash. This example suggests one way to cut calories without being hungry: Choose foods that take up a lot of space in your stomach compared with how many calories they have. Research shows that people decide when to stop eating a meal based on when their stomach is filled, not on when they've eaten a certain number of calories. When people or animals eat either an energy-dense meal or a less-dense meal, they eat about the same amount of food. As a result, they take in more calories when they eat an energy-dense meal.

Protein and carbohydrate have about 4 calories per gram. But fat has 9 calories per gram. As a result, high-fat foods are the densest in calories. For example, a single tablespoon of olive oil contains 119 calories. In contrast, a tablespoon of skim milk (which is almost all protein and carbohydrate) has only 11 calories.

Foods That Are High in Carbohydrates and Protein. Foods high in both carbohydrates and protein may help stave off hunger. Such foods include grains, beans, and dishes made with them (for example, spaghetti). Keep in mind, though, that carbohydrates affect your glucose level.

How to Do It. Here are some ways to include more high-fiber, low-calorie, high-carbohydrate foods in your day.

- Use brown rice instead of white rice.

- Use meat as the sideshow, not the main attraction. For example, if you like beef, serve it in stews, stir-fries, casseroles, and other dishes in which it takes second billing.

- Eat high-fiber cereals for breakfast.

- Eat fruits raw and in solid form, when possible. Juices have little fiber, and canning reduces the fiber as well. To eat more fresh fruits, try eating fresh fruits with breakfast, for snacks, and as dessert at lunch and dinner.

- Eat some vegetables raw. Cooking and canning lower the fiber content. To eat more raw vegetables, serve salad with lunch or dinner, or try vegetable sticks with a yogurt dip in place of chips and dip when watching TV.

- Choose low-fat breads (most bagels, buns, and loaves) more often than high-fat breads (croissants, biscuits, muffins, and cheese bread, for example). To eat more breads, try munching breadsticks for snacks, have toast or a bagel with your breakfast, serve rolls often with lunch and dinner, or serve sandwiches for meals.

- Increase the amount of rice or pasta and decrease the amount of topping.

- Substitute whole-wheat flour for a quarter to half of the amount of white flour needed when baking.

- Invest in some cookbooks that focus on nutritious foods you'd like to eat more of. These might include cookbooks for bread, beans, pasta, grains, or vegetables. Today, there is a wide range of low-fat cookbooks, from fast and easy to gourmet.

- Add a bit of wheat germ when making bread and casseroles. ("A bit" can range from a tablespoon to 1/2 cup, depending on how much you like the crunch and nutty flavor of wheat germ.)

- Serve soups often for meals. Because of their high liquid content, they are usually not dense in calories. (But watch out for cream soups!)

The Filling Meal

Changing the habits and atmosphere of your meals can also be helpful.

- Eat slowly. Give your brain time to get the news that you're full. To help eat more slowly, play slow music in the background, or put your fork down between bites.

- Focus your attention on the food and enjoy every bite. If you watch TV while eating or if you eat standing in the kitchen, it's easy to overeat without knowing it, and you won't even enjoy the food.

- Drink liquids with your meals and snacks.

- Set your place with a small plate or bowl. The first clue your brain gets about the size of your meal is from your eyes. Make it look big.

- Drop out of the Clean Plate Club. Eat what you are hungry for, then stop.

- Eat foods you like. Remember, healthful eating is not a punishment, but part of a gift—a longer, happier life—you give yourself.

- Put only half as much food on your plate as you usually eat. When you finish, think about whether you're still hungry. Only take seconds if you don't feel satisfied.

- Eat four or five small meals a day, if you're inclined and your schedule lets you. Eating small meals more often is actually better for your glucose levels than having just three meals a day. It also helps you feel less hungry.

The Flavorful Meal

Because fat carries flavor, low-fat cooking requires that you find other ways to punch up the flavor.

Herbs and Spices. Many plants have a strong scent or taste. Around the world, people use flavoring agents from plants to make their food tastier. The two main kinds of flavoring agents are herbs and spices.

Herbs are the leaves, flowers, and stems of flavoring plants. Parsley, sage, rosemary, and thyme are well-known herbs. Others are bay leaves, basil, oregano, mint, and dill. Herbs can be used fresh or dried.

Spices are the roots, seeds, and nuts of flavoring plants. Most spices are dried before use. These include cinnamon, cloves, poppy seeds, sesame seeds, cumin seeds, nutmeg, and black pepper. Others, such as ginger and garlic, may be used dried or fresh. Some "spices" are actually mixes of several spices. Curry powder and chili powder are two examples.

To use herbs and spices to flavor low-fat foods:

- Roast spices before adding to savory dishes to intensify the flavor.

- Buy whole spices instead of ground, and grind them yourself right before using.

- Buy fresh herbs instead of dried when you can. If a recipe calls for a certain amount of dried herbs, use triple that amount of fresh herbs. (Don't try this with spices, though. You'll change the character of the dish if you try to use fresh spices when a recipe calls for dried.)

- Increase the amount of spices by 50% if you remove a lot of fat from a baked dessert recipe.

- Don't let jarred herbs and spices sit around for years. They lose their flavor. Replace them with fresh every year or two if you haven't used them up.

- Think about starting a small herb garden outside your kitchen door. Or see if you can fit a few small plants on your windowsill. You'll always have a way of adding lots of flavor to food.

Other Flavor Enhancers. Herbs and spices are not the only way to add flavor to food.

- Sometimes marinate food before grilling or baking. Use a nonfat base such as wine or juice, and then add herbs, onion, or garlic.

- Choose recipes with strong-flavored ingredients. Chilies, mustard, vinegar, lemon juice, and horseradish are examples of ingredients with intense flavors.

- Double the amount of vanilla or other extracts when adapting a baked dessert recipe to be very low fat.

- Use only 100% real vanilla and other extracts in low-fat baking. Artificial flavors taste even more fake in low-fat baked goods than in regular ones.

- When you do use a high-fat ingredient, choose one with an intense flavor. For example, a small bit of aged Gruyère or cured Greek olives may add more flavor than a much larger amount of American cheese or canned olives.

- Choose the freshest fruits and vegetables with the brightest colors. These are likely to have the most flavor.

- Use cooking methods that intensify flavors. Roasting and grilling enhance not only meats but also onions, garlic, peppers, eggplants, and other vegetables.

EXPLORING NEW FOODS

In one way, changing diets is easy for Americans. Our citizens come from all over the world. So it's easy to learn about eating habits of other countries—just ask friends and neighbors of different ethnic backgrounds, go to your neighborhood Afghan or Vietnamese restaurant, or browse the cookbook section at your library.

A NEW PERSPECTIVE ON FOOD

"When I was dieting, I was always looking forward to getting off the diet so I could eat," says Elizabeth Zeno. "I assumed that everybody lived that way. I didn't realize that people aren't preoccupied with food the way I was. Before I went on this program, I knew everything in my cupboard and my refrigerator."

"This program" is a multipronged weight-loss program that involved consultation with many experts, taking weight-loss drugs, becoming more active, and learning new ways to think about food. Zeno no longer thinks about food all the time, and she has lost more than 70 pounds. "It's been fascinating to see the changes in me," she says. "I get up from the table when I'm full and just leave."

She has also become skilled at following the Food Guide Pyramid. For a long time, she kept food charts, counted both calories and grams, and measured her portions. "I wanted this information so ingrained in me that I could identify a cup of something or 3 ounces of something without ever having to hesitate," she says.

"This is the first time I've ever been on anything that it doesn't seem like a diet," Zeno says. "Now I feel like this is just a way of life."

Other cultures can give ideas for cutting back on meats and increasing the plant foods. To get you started, here are some dinner ideas from a variety of cultures. Although recipes for high-fat versions abound, all of these dishes can be tasty when made with little fat and little or no meat.

Grain Plus Vegetable. Most Americans already know and love spaghetti and other pasta dishes with a tomato or other vegetable sauce. Other grain and vegetable combinations include Chinese stir-fried vegetables over rice, Indian curries over rice, North African couscous, Lebanese tabbouleh, Spanish rice, and Mexican tortillas dipped in salsa.

Bean Plus Grain. One of the world's most widespread food combinations is beans and grains. Some examples you might try include New Orleans red beans and rice; American South Hoppin' John (black-eyed peas and rice); Cuban black beans and rice; Brazilian feijoada (black beans and rice); Egyptian kosheri and Indian kitchree (both are lentil and rice mixtures); Mexican bean tacos, burritos, and enchiladas; Middle Eastern hummus (chickpea spread) on pita bread; and Chinese stir-fried tofu over rice.

Bean Plus Grain Plus Vegetable. Some of the great soups of Europe are based on combining beans, grains, and vegetables, all in one pot. Examples include French pistou and Italian minestrone and pasta e fagioli.

WHAT TO DO ABOUT EATING OUT

Eating out does not have to mean abandoning your good habits. Here are some tips for making good choices at restaurants.

- Call the restaurant in advance and ask about the menu. Does it offer heart-healthy or low-calorie entrées? How about meat-free ones?

- Avoid all-you-can-eat places.

- Look for the "healthy" or "light" items. Some menus indicate low-fat dishes with hearts or other symbols.

- Skip items advertised as jumbo, giant, or deluxe.

- If you choose meat, go for broiled, roasted, grilled, or baked meats. Avoid fried meats.

- Ask the server what's in the dishes and how they're prepared.

- Ask the server if the kitchen will prepare special requests. For example, ask whether you can have your trout broiled instead of fried or have the skin removed from your chicken. Or ask whether you can have a green vegetable instead of the french fries that come with the meal.

- Be creative. You can often make a great meal out of soup, side dishes, or appetizers.

- Choose vegetables that are raw, stewed, steamed, or boiled. Avoid those in cream, cheese, or mayonnaise sauces.

- Get a small book that lists fat grams and calories that you can carry with you. You can then quickly check the fat or calorie content of foods on the menu or at the salad bar.

- Ask for salad dressings, gravies, sour cream, and sauces to be left off or served on the side.

- If you go to a restaurant with someone else, consider sharing an appetizer, main course, or dessert instead of each eating one.

- If your food shows up with a breaded coating, peel it off.

- Cut all visible fat and skin off meats.

- Eat only as much as you would at home. If you feel guilty about leaving food, ask to take the leftovers home.

- Eat only the foods you like and leave the rest. Why take in calories and not even enjoy them?

- Skip dessert or choose a low-fat one such as a fruit sorbet. Four ounces of sorbet has fewer than 150 calories.

WHAT TO DO ABOUT HOLIDAYS AND PARTIES

Celebrations are many people's downfall. They may be proud of their good habits most of the time, but then find themselves chugging eggnog at the office Christmas party or taste-testing all 10 platters of deviled eggs at a covered-dish dinner.

A little bit of thought and planning can help prevent these events from being calorie disasters and ensure that you can enjoy holidays and parties.

The Big Picture

Thanksgiving comes only once a year. Anniversaries, too. There's no reason to berate yourself if you don't stick rigidly to your meal plan on very special days. A little straying every once in a while won't sink your weight-loss plan. You may just level off for a couple of days. And you can keep your glucose controlled on special days by exercising more that day or, if you take insulin, by adjusting your dose.

On the other hand, not all celebrations are special events. An office with many employees might have birthday cake every other week. Some people get invited to many Christmas parties each December. The tips below will help you stay on your meal plan in many party situations.

Tips for Parties

- Look over your meal plan ahead of time. If you're not on insulin, you might move some Starch and Fat Exchanges from breakfast and lunch to later in the day so that you can eat more than usual in the evening, yet stay within your meal-plan guidelines.

- Don't try to eat everything. Study the choices, decide which dishes look yummiest, and eat just small samples.

- Pay attention to the taste, aroma, and texture of what you're eating. Savor each bite.

- Choose goals you can meet. For example, don't plan not to eat any treats at all at the party. Instead, you might plan to drink the spiced cider instead of the eggnog and to limit your dessert eating to just one or two spoonfuls.

- Part of the joy of celebrations is being with people you like. Focus on the people, not the food. For example, make a goal to talk with everyone in the room.

- Don't park yourself next to the food table. Stand at the opposite side of the room so that it takes some effort to get seconds.

- If the party is at your house, serve only healthful, filling foods. Most people won't even notice. Examples of foods that will please many people are low-fat pretzels, vegetables with a low-fat dip, fruit chunks, bread sticks, pickles, tossed salad, noodle salad, and sliced turkey breast.

- If the party is somewhere else, ask if you can bring a dish. Then there will be at least one low-fat food to eat.

- Volunteer to help. It's hard to eat when you're on a ladder hanging balloons.

- Beforehand, practice saying, "No, thank you." Have the phrase on the tip of your tongue in case your hosts pressure you to eat something.

The Skinny on Chapter

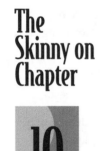

▶ You can eat a healthful, low-fat diet and still enjoy life.

▶ For you to stick to healthful eating habits for the rest of your life, your meals have to be filling and tasty.

▶ Foods that have a lot of fiber tend to make people feel full.

▶ Foods that are not calorie dense (that is, bulky, low-calorie foods) help keep you satisfied with fewer calories.

▶ Traditional diets of many cultures tend to be lower in fat and calories and higher in fiber than modern Western cuisine. So foreign cuisines can be a good source of tasty, low-calorie menu ideas.

▶ You don't have to fall off the wagon when you go to a party or restaurant. By planning ahead, you can stay within or close to your meal-plan goals.

An Active Lifestyle Helps Lost Pounds Stay Lost.

4

A healthful, reduced-calorie food plan can take pounds off, but many people gradually gain back the weight. And that brings us to the fourth key to successful weight loss: Exercise combined with healthful eating can combat the tendency for lost pounds to return. Exercise has other good benefits. An active lifestyle cuts your risk of heart disease, builds strong bones, and improves your outlook on life. An extra bonus is that exercise can improve glucose levels in people with type 2 diabetes. These chapters will help you get started on a more active life.

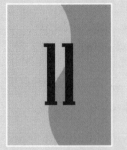

Fit for Living

I
f exercise could be bottled, it would be the perfect product to be hawked on late-night TV. "It can make your life easier in many ways! It can strengthen your lungs and heart so that you have more energy for everything you do! It may improve your mood! And it can reduce your risk for many diseases!"

But, unlike some of the products peddled on TV, exercise really can deliver on these promises. This chapter will fill you in on many ways that exercise can improve your life.

PSYCHOLOGICAL BENEFITS OF EXERCISE

A lot of anecdotes suggest that exercise can help your mental state.

- Aerobic exercise (exercise that strengthens your heart and lungs) may make you feel happier by changing your body chemistry.

- Exercise, especially aerobic exercise, may make you feel calmer.

- Exercise can brighten your mood by distracting you from pain and worries.

135

- Just as with any new skill you master, learning to exercise can improve your self-image.

- By helping you control your blood glucose, exercise helps your brain stay in the range of glucose levels where it works best.

- When your troubles or pains weigh down on you, exercise may take your mind off what is bothering you.

If your weight has been holding you back from what you want to do, then exercising will give you back the ability to do many things. When you

END OF ONE LIFE, START OF ANOTHER

"My bullet-proof, carefree, do-as-you-will lifestyle as I perceived it had been dealt a swift death blow," says Luke Lewis, describing his reaction to getting diabetes.

He had suspected diabetes already. He had researched his symptoms—including frequent urination, thirstiness, and vision problems—on the World Wide Web. An endocrinologist confirmed his fears.

"I have always felt that knowledge is power," Lewis says. "My days and nights were filled with research on subjects such as biochemistry, nutrition, the endocrine system, chemistry, metabolism, and neurotransmitters."

Lewis says that he went through an intense self-assessment and composed a plan of action. "I'm a goal-oriented person," he says. "I felt that this was an opportune time to do something about my sedentary lifestyle and resultant obesity." He was spurred on by additional online explorations, which had taken him to an Internet diabetes support group. There he heard about people who had not acted in time to control their diabetes and were suffering complications. So he decided to take "a proactive stance towards my health in general." Diet and exercise have now brought his diabetes under good control, and he plans to continue them forever.

become fit enough to spend the afternoon shopping or walking around a museum, just as normal-weight people can, the freedom will make you feel on top of the world.

HEALTH BENEFITS OF EXERCISE

How exercise affects people mentally is still somewhat fuzzy. Not so the good physical effects. Research clearly shows that exercise can improve your health, including your diabetes, and lengthen your life. (See the box "Spotlight on Research: When Habits Change.")

General Health Benefits

Chapter 4 described the many diseases associated with overweight and how losing weight can reduce your risk of disease. Many of those same diseases are linked to inactivity. Becoming more active can help you be healthier, just as losing weight can.

One good effect is that exercise lowers people's risk of heart and blood vessel disease. This occurs because exercise is thought to:

- Lower blood pressure

- Protect against the artery-clogging effects of cholesterol

- Raise levels of good (HDL) cholesterol

- Improve circulation

- Reduce the number of blood clots

These effects on the heart and blood vessels are extra important for people with diabetes, who are more likely than other people to get diseases of these organs.

Exercise also appears to reduce the risk of colon cancer and perhaps some other cancers as well. Exercise can improve how well people with osteoarthritis or rheumatoid arthritis function in their daily lives. And exercise builds strong bones, slowing down the weakening of bone that occurs as people, especially women, get older.

SPOTLIGHT ON RESEARCH
When Habits Change

Good health and exercise go hand in hand, so you can't be certain in many studies which causes the other. That is, people who are healthy may be more likely to exercise than other people. One study that takes into account this relationship is the Aerobics Center Longitudinal Study.

In the Aerobics Center Longitudinal Study, researchers looked at 25,341 men and 7,080 women who had a preventative health exam at the Cooper Clinic in Dallas, Texas, between 1970 and 1989. All participants took a treadmill test at their first exam to find out how fit they were.

According to results published in the *Journal of the American Medical Association* in 1996, the people in the bottom fifth of fitness were significantly more likely to die during the study. This higher risk appeared whether the people were in good health or whether they had other health problems, such as high blood pressure, diabetes, or smoking. In fact, people who were in good health but were inactive had higher death rates than active people with health problems.

Other results from this study, published a year earlier in the *Journal of the American Medical Association,* described 9,777 men who had at least two preventative exams during the study period. The study's goal was to see how changes in physical fitness affected mortality. The men were divided into two groups: healthy men and men who had had certain health problems such as heart attacks, stroke, diabetes, or high blood pressure.

Some men were fit at both exams, some were unfit at both, and some became more fit or less fit during the study. Men who were fit both times had the lowest death rates. Those who were unfit at both exams had the highest death rates. Men who started out unfit but then became fit had a lower death rate than men who stayed unfit. These results were true for both healthy men and those with health problems.

This study shows it's never too late to get started on better fitness. Even if you already have diabetes or high blood pressure, odds are that better fitness will improve your life.

Exercise and Diabetes

Exercise helps people with type 2 diabetes in at least four ways:

- It brings blood glucose down for awhile. Regular exercise can thus help with long-term control.

- Exercise may make cells more responsive to insulin.

- Diabetes puts people at extra risk of heart disease. Exercise helps improve cholesterol levels and lower blood pressure.

- Exercise can help with losing weight and keeping it off.

People with diabetes who want to begin an exercise program should talk first to their doctors. They should also follow the safety tips in Chapter 12.

The box "Spotlight on Research: Medical Outcomes Study" shows some of the benefits of exercise for people with diabetes.

Exercise and Your Life Span

Exercise can even help people live longer. At least, that's the message of some long-running studies of exercise and health.

For example, in the Harvard Alumni Study, researchers have followed men who entered Harvard University from 1916 through 1950. The men received physicals when they started college. Every so often, the research team sends them questionnaires to fill out about their health and exercise habits.

In a 1986 article in the *New England Journal of Medicine*, the researchers reported that the more active the men, the lower their risk of death. For example, men who walked more than 3 miles a week were substantially less likely to die than men who walked less than that. The older a man was, the more physical activity helped. For example, for men between 70 and 84, those who burned more than 2,000 calories a week in physical activities had half the death rate of men who burned less than 500. For men between 35 and 49, burning 2,000 calories reduced the death rate by about 21%. According to a 1994 report in *Medicine and*

Science in Sports and Exercise, it did not matter whether the men had played sports in college. If a Harvard grad was currently active, then he had a lower risk of death.

The Harvard Alumni Study shows that the more active a man is, the longer on average he lives. It also suggests that the good effects of exercise don't get stored up. Men who started exercising in middle age benefited as much from their exercise as men who had exercised for years. And exercise can help older people as well.

This study and others like it make a strong case that people who exercise and become more fit live longer.

SPOTLIGHT ON RESEARCH
Medical Outcomes Study

The Medical Outcomes Study is a long-term study of health-care systems in Boston, Chicago, and Los Angeles. In a report in the *Journal of Clinical Epidemiology* in 1994, researchers used 2 years of data from the Medical Outcomes Study to see whether being active improves the lives of people with diabetes and other chronic illnesses. The subjects were 1,758 adults with high blood pressure, diabetes, heart disease, or depression. The researchers looked at their mental and physical well-being and how active they were at the beginning of the study and after 2 years.

Both at the beginning of the study and at the end, people who were physically active functioned better. For example, at the end of the study, the people who exercised more had fewer limitations in physical and social activities, more energy, fewer sleep problems, and less depression and anxiety.

This study shows that the benefits of exercise are not limited to healthy people. People who have serious medical conditions but are active anyway tend to feel better in both body and mind.

The Skinny on Chapter

▶ Exercise can distract you from pain or problems and improve your self-image.

▶ Exercise can reduce the chance of many diseases, including heart and blood vessel diseases, colon cancer, and osteoporosis.

▶ Exercise can improve glucose levels in people with type 2 diabetes.

▶ People who are physically fit tend to live longer, even if they have other health problems.

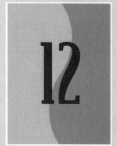

Getting Started on an Active Life

I f you're like many people with diabetes, your health care team has probably suggested that you exercise. You may feel as lost as if you had been told to start a yak farm or to collect amphoras glazed in Attic black. You're likely to have plenty of questions. How? Why? When? How often? Can I afford it? And how do I go about choosing the yaks (or jars, or exercises), anyway? Even if you have exercised before, starting again now that you're older and have diabetes can be scary.

There are many options today to suit a variety of bodies and personalities. This chapter will help you find ways to put more exercise in your life. It will explain the different kinds of exercise and what they do for you. You will also learn how to stay safe when you exercise.

BECOMING MORE ACTIVE

In Chapter 13, you'll learn how much exercise you need to do and how to measure how much you're doing. You may be surprised at your options and how sometimes even a little exercise can have big effects. You'll see that:

142

- Being a little active is better than not being active at all.

- Being more active is usually better than being less active.

Almost everyone can benefit from making the effort to sit less and move more. Exercise does not have to be strenuous to be useful. In fact, moving any part of your body is considered exercise by many experts.

Even if you are a very busy person, you can probably squeeze more activity into your schedule. The box "Ways to Get Moving" lists small changes that people can make in their lives to become more active. Some may work for you.

TWO KINDS OF EXERCISE: AEROBIC AND RESISTANCE

Doctors generally divide exercise into two types. One is aerobic exercise. This is exercise that strengthens your heart and lungs. When these organs are strong, you have more endurance. You can work longer before getting tired.

The other kind of exercise is resistance (strength training). This is exercise that works muscles so they become stronger. With a good strength-training program, a person gains flexibility, balance, and coordination.

In some ways, resistance training prepares you to put out a burst of strength for brief, quick activities (such as picking up a bag of groceries or hitting a baseball). Aerobic training prepares you to endure long-lasting activities. Such activities include long-distance swimming and running. More practically, aerobic training may help you do house chores without rest breaks, last through a long day of rushing from meeting to meeting, or host a child's birthday party.

Both the lung-strengthening and the muscle-strengthening aspects of exercise are important. The best exercise program includes both aerobic and resistance activities.

Getting Aerobically Fitter

It's easy to recognize an exercise that challenges your aerobic fitness. When you do it, you breathe harder, and your heart beats faster. If you keep it up for 20 minutes or more, you are strengthening your heart and lungs. These exercises also burn lots of calories and so work well for keeping you from gaining weight. (Chapter 13 will discuss in detail how much aerobic exercise you should do.)

WAYS TO GET MOVING

- Take the stairs, not the elevator.

- Park at the far end of the parking lot and walk to where you're going.

- Hide the remote control and get up to change channels.

- Use a rake instead of a leaf blower.

- Get off the bus or subway a few blocks early and finish your trip by foot.

- Use an old-fashioned, nonpolluting push reel mower instead of a powered mower.

- Walk around while you talk on the phone.

- When you plan a get-together with friends or family, choose activities such as dancing, bowling, or skating. If cultural activities are more your style, try going to a museum or taking a walking tour.

- Dance at weddings.

- Stand instead of sitting when you can, such as when you give dictation, file, sharpen pencils, use a calculator, or chop vegetables.

- Walk your dog an extra time or two every day.

- Wash your car by hand instead of going to the carwash.

- Use your lunch hour and coffee breaks to walk for a few minutes. If you eat lunch out, don't always choose the closest restaurant.

- Don't automatically sit down in front of the TV every night. If none of your favorite shows are on, think about doing something: working in your yard or going to the mall or walking to the park to swing on the swings.

WAYS TO GET MOVING *Continued*

- If you do watch TV, do something else at the same time. You could iron, sort bills and papers, dust, straighten up, sort laundry, ride a stationary bicycle, or polish shoes, for example.

- Get up during commercials and walk around.

- Walk to business meetings instead of catching a taxi.

- Vacuum your rugs and carpets as often as the manufacturer suggests.

- March in a parade.

- Start a hobby that will get you moving around, such as gardening or golfing.

- Move your telephones at home and work so that you will have to get up from the sofa or your desk to answer them.

- Walk to the mailbox instead of driving.

Aerobic exercises come in many shapes, sizes, and flavors. Because there are so many types, people who want to start exercising can usually find some aerobic activity that appeals to them. Here are some examples:

- Cycling on a stationary bicycle

- Cross-country skiing

- Chopping wood

- Vigorous dancing (such as waltzes, polkas, and swing dances)

- Aerobics classes

- Walking briskly

Getting Stronger

Strong muscles make your life easier. They'll help you open those heavy doors at the post office, load cat litter into your grocery cart, and pick up a tired toddler.

The main way to build strength is through weight lifting. You can literally "lift weights" by using dumbbells and barbells. Or you can use a resistance exercise machine. You'll often see these at health clubs, and some are available for home use as well. You can buy stretchy rubber exercise bands. Or you can raid your pantry for cans of vegetables (1 pound apiece) and jugs of water (about 8 pounds). No matter what you use, the principle is the same: You need to make the muscle work hard. (Chapter 13 discusses how much resistance exercise you should do.)

Can Everyone Do Weight Training? Men and women alike can benefit from resistance exercise. Women who do muscle training get stronger, just as men do. Muscle is muscle, no matter whom it's in. And strength depends in part on neural factors: Your nerves may start to work together better, and you may learn not to hold yourself back. Because resistance exercise helps build sturdy bones, it can help prevent osteoporosis, which women are more likely to get than men. So as women get older, strength training becomes more important.

Similarly, both young and old people can benefit from weight training. In fact, strength training is especially good for older people. People tend to lose muscle as they age. A strengthening program helps thwart this decline. Strong muscles let older people get around easier by helping them with walking, climbing stairs, and other activities they do every day. Strong muscles may also help people avoid falls by improving balance, agility, and coordination.

Some older people may have health problems that prevent them from exercising. For example, people who have trouble keeping their balance, have high blood pressure, or have hardening of the arteries in the brain may be advised by their doctors not to exercise. So like anyone else with diabetes, older people with diabetes should talk to their doctor before starting an exercise program.

Weight Training and Weight Loss. Resistance exercise doesn't burn as many calories as aerobic exercise. But resistance exercise should be part of your exercise program anyway. Getting stronger will make almost every activity in your life easier. And it may boost your energy.

STRETCHING

It's not aerobic. It's not muscle building. Even so, stretching has a place in everyone's fitness program.

First, stretching gets you moving your muscles and body. If you're not in good shape, stretching can prepare you mentally for starting an exercise program.

Second, stretching makes you more flexible. You are then less likely to injure yourself. You can do more. You may become more graceful.

Third, stretching can help you relax. For that reason, it may reduce pain caused by tight muscles.

AN EXERCISE SMORGASBORD

One thing that should be clear is that exercise should always be tailored to **you.** The one-size-fits-all approach of your grade-school days—when the gym teacher demanded that each kid do the same number of sit-ups or jumping jacks—just isn't suitable. Both aerobic exercise and resis-

SPOTLIGHT ON RESEARCH
Exercise and the Elderly

One study of the value of exercise for elderly people was the Frailty and Injuries: Cooperative Studies of Intervention Techniques (known by the optimistic nickname FICSIT). According to a report in the *New England Journal of Medicine* in 1994, Boston researchers put 100 people who lived in a nursing home either on a resistance-training program or not. These people ranged in age from 72 to 98. After 10 weeks of doing knee- and hip-strengthening exercises every other day, men and women in the exercise group greatly improved their leg strength. They could walk faster and climb stairs better. But those who were not in the exercise group changed little in 10 weeks.

The FICSIT study shows that even people who are frail and quite old can build muscle.

tance exercise require that you push yourself to do more than you usually do, while not trying to do more than is possible. This point is different for each person and changes as you get stronger and fitter.

People's personalities also differ. Some people prefer to do things by themselves. Others prefer to exercise socially. Some people want to compete with themselves. Others prefer to compete against some external standard. Choosing activities that you'll enjoy is very important. If you don't, it will be hard to stay with them.

Following are several exercises that are well suited for beginners. All can be done at an easy level or a harder level. All are fairly safe. And most don't require a lot of costly equipment.

Walking

Walking is one of the best exercises there is. It is also one of the most fun exercises because you can choose whatever scenery you will enjoy the most—anything from stores at the mall to fancy houses in the ritzy part of town to country vistas. (Some malls open their doors early so that people can get in some walking time before work.) It's suitable for people of all ages. And it's cheap, too. All you need is a good pair of walking shoes.

Bicycling or Stationary Cycling

Like walking, bicycling offers lots of choices of scenery and is something you already know how to do and can do with friends or relatives. It does require more equipment than most beginner exercises. In addition to a decent bicycle, you'll also want a bicycle helmet and some equipment, such as a water bottle. If you prefer a stationary bicycle, you can get some good exercise while catching up on the news. And you can do it in any weather. Bicycling is mostly an aerobic exercise.

Swimming

Swimming can be as strenuous as you desire. Yet it is gentle on the joints, even in people who are heavy or have arthritis or back problems. If you have access to an indoor pool, swimming is an exercise you can do year-round. Men burn more calories than women during swimming because they are less buoyant and so must put more energy into staying afloat.

Water Aerobics

Water aerobics are calisthenics done in the pool. Compared with aerobics on land, water aerobics are less stressful on the joints. Because of water's buoyancy, even heavy people can jump high and leap gracefully. You don't need to know how to swim to do water aerobics. Call local pools and recreation centers to find a class. Despite its name, water aerobics offers both aerobic and resistance benefits.

Yoga

Hatha yoga (the most popular form of yoga) combines motions, meditation, and structured breathing. The goals are to increase strength and flexibility and reduce stress. It can easily be adapted to people with special needs, such as those in wheelchairs. It's best to start by taking a class rather than trying to learn from a book or video. Yoga is a strength-building exercise.

EXERCISE PRECAUTIONS

Every activity in life carries some risk. Exercise is no exception. Even people who are in perfect health can injure themselves exercising.

Staying Safe

The health risks of exercise often involve doing things too long or too hard or with too little attention. Ways to avoid most of these risks are:

- Start slowly. Don't go straight from couch potato to running an hour every day.

- Avoid high-impact activities (such as jogging and skipping rope) when you first start an exercise program.

- Spread your exercise throughout the week. Don't exercise just on weekends.

- Warm up before starting to exercise. Warm-ups should start with a light aerobic activity and then proceed to a stretching activity. Examples of warm-up aerobic exercises include walking and calisthenics. Or you can practice an action taken from your sport (for example, throwing a ball around before a ball game). Warm-up exercise is believed to reduce injuries. It helps you turn your attention to what you are about to do. By stretching out your muscles, it may also make them resist injury better. It's also good to do similar activities to cool down after you exercise.

- Strengthen vulnerable joints. For example, if you want to play tennis, stretching and strengthening exercises for your shoulder and elbow can help them resist injuries. If you want to run, focus on strengthening and stretching ankles and knees.

- Breathe. Holding your breath during exercises can make your blood pressure shoot up.

- Drink plenty of water when exercising.

- Be aware of risks, and keep an eye out for them.

- Stop if you get shaky or if pain starts.

- Choose practical exercise clothes. They should keep you from getting too hot or too cold. They should also allow you to move easily without tripping you or catching on equipment.

- Use appropriate, well-fitting safety equipment. For example, wear a helmet when bicycling. Make sure your shoes fit well and are suitable for the sport.

- Check over exercise equipment before using it.

- Practice good technique. For example, if you are lifting weights, use the proper stance, breathe properly, and lift and lower with the correct motions. For some exercises, such as tennis and golf, lessons may be a wise investment at the start.

- Choose a forgiving exercise surface. Dirt and grass cushion your movements and don't hurt as much if you fall. Wood, cinders, and asphalt are gentler than cement. Exercise shoes should be well cushioned inside.

Special Precautions for People With Diabetes

People with diabetes need to take a little extra care when exercising.

- First and foremost, always talk to your doctor before starting an exercise program! This is extra important for people over 40, but everyone with diabetes should do it. Depending on what complications of diabetes (or other diseases) you have or are at extra risk of getting, your doctor may steer you toward certain exercises and away from others. For example, if you have diabetic eye disease, your doctor may advise you not to lift weights or do certain yoga poses. If you've lost feeling in your feet, your doctor may not want you to take up running or jogging. Also, exercise will affect your glucose levels, and your doctor can give you advice about whether you'll need to adjust your drug dose or snack schedule.

- Wear good foot gear. The shoes should match your activity. Like any shoes you choose, they should be smooth inside and fit well. Your socks should always be clean and seam-free and made of polyester or a cotton-polyester blend.

- Check your feet after every exercise session. Make sure that they are unharmed, with no blisters, cuts, cracks, or other sores.

- Test your glucose level before exercising and again afterward. Don't exercise if your glucose level is more than 300 mg/dl. Also don't exercise if your glucose is greater than 250 mg/dl and you have ketones in your urine. If your glucose level is less than 100 mg/dl, have a snack containing about 15 grams of carbohydrate (such as 4 ounces of orange juice, 2 teaspoons

of sugar, or five to seven hard candies) and test again before
exercising.

- Keep track of your glucose readings so that you'll learn how
  exercise affects your glucose level.

- Be prepared for a low-blood-glucose reaction (also called
  hypoglycemia or an insulin reaction) during and after exercise. If you use insulin or sulfonylurea diabetes pills, exercise
  may lower your glucose level too much. Have your glucose
  meter on hand so you can test during exercise. Also have a

CRISIS AT THE MALL

"Exercise is the foundation for all diets," says Juanita Diaz. She
tries to live an active life, but finds balancing exercise with her
insulin regimen tricky.

She remembers one crisis in particular. "My sugar dropped so
fast," says Diaz. "I was on one of my low-calorie diets. I had eaten
my supper and taken my medication, and I had walked down to the
mall with the children and we walked around." But suddenly, her
glucose level plummeted. She got shaky and started sweating. "It was
so scary."

Luckily, she had trained her boys well. They saw her sweating and
shaking and forced her to eat some food. They were also prepared if
her insulin reaction had worsened. "They know how to give a shot
of [glucagon] if I ever should get into a coma," she says.

After her insulin reaction at the mall, Diaz's husband was con-
cerned and upset. "He said, 'You need to eat more food if you're
going to walk,'" she says. She protested that she had eaten supper,
and that a similar trip to the mall the day before was uneventful. As
best as she can guess, walking just a little more than usual caused
her crisis. One of her reasons for wanting to lose weight is to get off
insulin and not have to worry about low-blood-glucose reactions
anymore.

source of glucose (a tube of cake icing, glucose tablets, raisins, or other source of sugar) with you to treat a reaction. Don't keep exercising during a reaction.

- Plan your exercise around your meal schedule and insulin schedule. Your doctor will probably suggest that you exercise 1 to 3 hours after eating because the risk of low blood glucose will be less then. If you take insulin, it's best not to exercise when it is working its hardest. Your doctor can tell you when that is. It's also best not to exercise just before going to bed.

- Talk to your doctor to learn whether to alter your insulin dose when you exercise and if so, precisely how to do so.

- If you exercise more than an hour, have a snack every 30 to 60 minutes.

- Wear an I.D. necklace, bracelet, or shoe tag that says you have diabetes.

- Drink water before, during, and after exercise. One cup of water every 20 minutes is about right for many people. If you weigh less after exercising than before, you're not drinking enough.

- Don't exercise outside when it's very hot or very cold. Choose indoor activities on those days.

- If you take an exercise class, tell the teacher you have diabetes.

- For exercising in water, choose a pool whose temperature is in the low 80°s.

- Report any strange symptoms during or after exercise to your doctor.

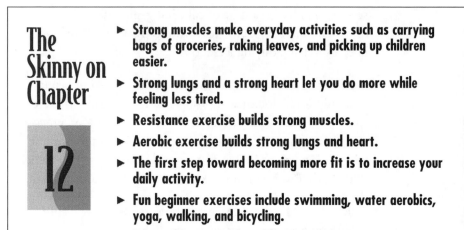

The Skinny on Chapter

12

► Strong muscles make everyday activities such as carrying bags of groceries, raking leaves, and picking up children easier.

► Strong lungs and a strong heart let you do more while feeling less tired.

► Resistance exercise builds strong muscles.

► Aerobic exercise builds strong lungs and heart.

► The first step toward becoming more fit is to increase your daily activity.

► Fun beginner exercises include swimming, water aerobics, yoga, walking, and bicycling.

► Take safety precautions when exercising.

► People with diabetes need to measure their blood glucose levels before and after exercise—and sometimes during, as well.

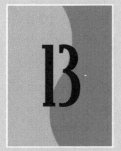

It takes less exercise than you think to reduce your risk of disease, make you stronger, and improve your glucose control.

How Much Exercise You Need

Exercise myths are everywhere. "If it doesn't hurt, it's not doing you any good," one person advises you. "You gotta sweat!" says another. "It's not supposed to be fun! It's good for you," says a third.

It's no wonder many people shy away from exercise. All too often, people think of exercise as something painful and stinky that consumes their free time and requires getting shoved around on a ball court.

But the scientific evidence says something different. Sure, exercise is good for your health. Sure, the more you do, the better it usually is. But exercise does not have to be unpleasant or steal all your personal time to help your health. It doesn't even have to be vigorous. This chapter will show you how to exercise for better health or fitness.

THE SURGEON GENERAL'S REPORT

Physical Activity and Health: A Report of the Surgeon General is a government report released in 1996. Dozens of scientists examined hundreds of scientific studies to learn the effects of exercise on health. They also reviewed the exercise recommendations of a dozen organizations, including the Centers for

Disease Control, the American College of Sports Medicine, and the American Heart Association.

The report concluded that people can improve their health and quality of life by being moderately physically active for a total of about half an hour every day or nearly every day. Moderate physical activity—which includes activities you're probably already doing, such as raking leaves or mowing the grass—is healthful for young and old, male and female.

It's important to stress that the Surgeon General is not asking you to become a marathon runner. People who change from being sedentary to being a little active are doing themselves a lot of good.

The report offers the most comprehensive look at what exercise can do for you. It is the basis of many of the suggestions in this chapter.

HEALTH VS. FITNESS

Exercising for fitness and exercising for good health are not the same thing.

Being physically fit means that your everyday life poses no physical challenges for you. You can alertly and vigorously do what you have to without overtiring yourself. And you still have energy left over for having fun or dealing with emergencies. To get to this state of fitness, experts generally suggest that people spend 20 to 60 minutes doing aerobic exercise 3 to 5 days a week. This amount of physical exercise strengthens the heart and lungs for endurance.

Although being fit is a good goal for everyone, not everyone has the time or desire to do that much aerobic exercise. Exercising for health stresses instead keeping the organs and bones in good working order. Compared with exercising for fitness, exercising for health is less strenuous. But it takes more time and needs to be done more frequently. Even so, exercising for health is much easier to work into daily activities because you can do it in bits and pieces rather than needing to carve out big blocks of time.

EXERCISING FOR HEALTH: THE LEAST YOU CAN DO

To reduce your chances of diseases, your exercise program should have three components.

- It should contain endurance activities of "moderate intensity."

- You should follow it 5 to 7 days a week.

- It should total about 30 minutes per day.

In addition, most exercise guidelines suggest that people also do resistance exercises at least twice a week. These exercises should stress strengthening the largest muscles of the body.

The exercise you choose is up to you. It can be something you do special, outside your ordinary activities. Or it can be chores you'd be doing anyway. Or it can be something fun.

The 150-Calorie Rule

One definition of a day's worth of moderate activity is activity that burns 150 calories. Each of the following burns about 150 calories for an average 150-pound person (if you weigh less than 150 pounds, it will take you longer to burn 150 calories, but if you weigh more than 150 pounds, you will burn 150 calories faster):

- Washing and waxing a car for 45 to 60 minutes

- Washing windows or floors for 45 to 60 minutes

- Playing volleyball for 45 minutes

- Playing touch football for 30 to 45 minutes

- Gardening for 30 to 45 minutes

- Wheeling oneself in a wheelchair for 30 to 40 minutes

- Walking 1 3/4 miles in 35 minutes or 2 miles in 30 minutes

- Playing basketball for 15 to 20 minutes or shooting baskets for 30 minutes

- Bicycling 5 miles in 30 minutes or 4 miles in 15 minutes

- Dancing fast for 30 minutes

- Pushing a stroller 1 1/2 miles in 30 minutes

- Raking leaves for 30 minutes

- Doing water aerobics for 30 minutes

- Swimming laps for 20 minutes

- Playing wheelchair basketball for 20 minutes

- Jumping rope for 15 minutes

- Running 1 1/2 miles in 15 minutes

- Stairwalking for 15 minutes

More Personalized Measures of Moderate Exercise

Common sense says that moderate exercise means different things to a 20-year-old and to her 80-year-old grandmother or to an Olympic athlete and to someone whose 10-hour workday is spent at a desk. The activities listed above don't take differences in age, fitness, or health into account. You may find it more sensible to choose moderate exercise based on what is moderate for **you.**

One definition of moderate exercise is an exercise that gets your heart beating at about 50% to 70% of its maximum beating rate. To estimate your maximum heart rate, subtract your age from 220.

For example, if you are 50 years old, your maximum heart rate is probably about 170 (that is, 220 minus 50). To exercise moderately, you would want to get your heart beating between 85 and 119 beats per minute (50% to 70% of 170).

To tell how fast your heart is beating, take your pulse. You should be able to find your pulse at your wrist or where your jaw meets your neck. As you watch the second hand of a watch go around for 1 minute, count how many times your heart beats. Or count the beats in 15 seconds and multiply by 4. If you have trouble, your doctor or nurse can show you how to take your pulse.

Some people can't reliably estimate their maximum heart rate by subtracting their age from 220. For example, some blood pressure drugs lower a person's maximum heart rate. Diabetic nerve disease can sometimes change the heart rate as well. Such people need to use a different rule.

If you don't want to use your heart rate, try the conversation rule: If you are too out of breath to carry on a conversation, you're working too hard.

How Do I Get In 30 Minutes a Day?

The Surgeon General's guidelines say that it's okay to get your 30 minutes of exercise in bits and pieces. If you can squeeze in 8 minutes here and 10 minutes there, you can add them together.

If you have a busy life, finding even 5 spare minutes may seem hard. Here are some times you may be able to fit in a few minutes of walking or stair climbing:

- During television commercials

- During coffee breaks

- During lunch breaks

- While talking on a cellular phone

- While waiting for a subway train, a bus, or an airplane

- During intermission at a concert or half-time at a ball game

Also, there's always the option of doing two things at once. For example, if you usually read the paper in the morning before work, think about reading it while cycling on a stationary bicycle. After you park the car or get off the subway and are walking to your office, take a more roundabout route. If you're meeting a friend, walk around the park or a shopping mall instead of sitting in a café eating croissants.

Some people find it useful to schedule their exercise for a certain time each day. Then it becomes as much a part of the normal routine as eating, brushing teeth, watching the news, or washing dishes.

People With Diabetes

Even though an exercising-for-health program is not very strenuous, you still should not start up on your own. People with diabetes should always check with their doctors before starting to exercise. So should people with heart or blood vessel diseases, nerve disease, loss of feeling, or another chronic health problem. Your doctor can make sure you have chosen a program that won't overstress your heart or worsen your diabetes or complications.

In addition, people who are not used to exercise should start slowly and work up to 30 minutes a day. Remember, you're trying to learn healthful habits for the rest of your life. Overdoing it in the first week will just give you sore muscles and a reason to quit.

EXERCISING FOR FITNESS: A NEXT STEP

Exercising a total of 30 minutes every day may be the least you can do for health, but it's not the best you can do. Researchers believe that exercising to become fit can cut your risks of diseases even more. Unlike exercising for health, exercising for fitness will probably require you to set aside some special time for it.

To start to exercise for fitness, you can:

- Increase how hard you exercise (for example, shoot for 70% to 80% of your maximum heart rate)

- Increase how long you exercise at one time (at least 20 minutes per session and preferably longer)

- Increase how much you exercise each day (for example, walking for 1 hour instead of 1/2 hour)

Any of these steps will increase the number of calories you burn.

EXERCISING FOR STRENGTH

In a typical weight-lifting program, you lift a certain weight a certain number of times. As you get stronger, you make the weight heavier, but keep the number of lifts the same.

Experts do not agree on the precise number of times you should lift a weight. But in general, if you want to increase only your muscle endurance, you would lift a lighter weight more times (for example, choose a weight you can lift 15 to 20 times). To increase strength, lift a heavier weight fewer times (for example, choose a weight you can lift only

6 to 8 times). In a general-purpose program that would build both strength and endurance, you would choose something between these two extremes (for example, choose a weight you can lift only 8 to 12 times).

At first, do just one set of lifts. Later, if you want to increase your workout, you can do several sets of lifts, resting for a few minutes after completing each set. Experts also recommend that you allow at least 48 hours between weight-lifting sessions to give muscles time to rest. If you want to exercise more often than that, work on certain muscles one day and different muscles the next.

If you don't want to lift weights, some exercises can also make you stronger. You may remember many of these from long-ago gym classes. They include leg lifts, push-ups, and crunches (the modern, safer version of a sit-up). You can use giant rubber bands or springs or elastic tubes with some of these exercises to increase how much work your muscles are doing.

No matter whether you lift weights or do strengthening exercises, resistance training should focus on seven areas: legs, arms, hips, shoulders, abdomen, back, and chest.

EXERCISING FOR GOOD GLUCOSE CONTROL

The American Diabetes Association recommends that, to improve glucose levels, people with type 2 diabetes should exercise for 30 to 60 minutes at a time, three or four times a week. This exercise program should be moderate to hard. Each exercise session should start with 5 to 10 minutes of light aerobic exercise followed by 5 to 10 minutes of stretching. Each session should end with 5 to 10 minutes of cooldown exercises. Good cooldowns are low-intensity versions of whatever your exercise was—for example, after running, a good cooldown exercise is walking. And of course, people with type 2 diabetes should see their doctors before starting an exercise program.

What about people with type 1 diabetes? The American Diabetes Association position is that there is no evidence that exercise helps glucose levels in people with type 1 diabetes. But people with type 1 diabetes are encouraged to exercise to help their hearts and to have fun.

No matter what form of diabetes you have, you should carefully follow the safety tips in Chapter 12.

EXERCISING FOR WEIGHT LOSS

Exercising probably won't make you lose much weight. Yet it is one of the most valuable parts of your weight-loss plan. A contradiction? Not at all. It turns out that exercise helps to keep you from gaining weight. Once you lose weight, exercise is your best bet for keeping it off. (See the box "Spotlight on Research: Calorie Cutting vs. Exercise in Weight Loss.")

Why Exercise Helps

Differences between muscle and body fat explain both why you might not lose weight by exercise alone and why exercising helps keep pounds off.

First, exercise can be making you obviously trimmer and more fit, yet you may see little difference in your weight. Although you are losing fat, you are gaining muscle.

Second, even when you are watching TV or sleeping, your body is using energy. The more muscle you have, the more calories you burn all the time. So there are fewer unburned calories to end up as extra pounds.

Burning Calories

In theory, you must burn 3,500 calories to lose 1 pound. In real life, your body has ways of regulating your eating and activity patterns to keep its

SPOTLIGHT ON RESEARCH

Calorie Cutting vs. Exercise in Weight Loss

A study in the *Journal of the American Dietetic Association* in 1996 reveals the different roles of calorie cutting and exercise in weight loss. Young adults who were at least 31 pounds overweight volunteered for a 1-year-long obesity-treatment program. Forty-two people went on a reduced-calorie heart-healthy meal plan. Forty-three other people joined a walking program. Another 42 people ate the heart-healthy diet and also joined the walking program.

SPOTLIGHT ON RESEARCH *Continued*

The pattern of weight loss differed between groups:

- People who were on diet treatment alone lost an average of 15 pounds in the first 3 months. In general, they did not lose any more weight, and they began gaining weight again after the 1-year program was over. Two years after starting the weight-loss program, these people weighed 2 pounds more than when they started.

- People who only exercised lost weight slower and lost less of it—about 1 1/2 pounds after 3 months and 6 pounds after 1 year. But these people stayed at about that weight for the next year.

- People on the combination treatment had a weight-loss pattern that combined elements of the other two programs. Like the diet-only people, people in the combo group lost a good amount of weight in the first 3 months, but they regained weight after the end of the study. Like the exercise-only people, the combination-treatment people continued losing weight after 3 months. After 1 year, they had lost an average of almost 20 pounds. They then rebounded to a weight on average about 5 pounds below their starting weight.

This study shows clearly how diet and exercise have different effects on weight-loss patterns. People who included exercise in their weight-loss strategy had an easier time preventing weight regain than people who only cut calories. The results suggest that sticking with an exercise program was easier than sticking with a reduced-calorie food plan. Because a third of the volunteers dropped out in the first year and another third did not come in for the 2-year exam, group sizes became rather small. So these results will need to be confirmed by other studies.

weight even. But let's pretend that your body actually will lose 1 pound for every 3,500 calories you burn. Let's also pretend that you weigh 200 pounds. Then to lose 1 pound, you could:

- Play the flute for 18 1/4 hours

- Mop floors for 10 1/4 hours

- Play table tennis for 9 1/2 hours

- Golf for 7 1/2 hours

- Skateboard for 5 1/2 hours

- Do karate for 3 1/3 hours

For comparison's sake, it would take nearly 31 hours of sitting quietly to burn 3,500 calories. If you weigh less than 200 pounds, you would have to do these activities even longer to burn 3,500 calories.

If you weigh more than 200 pounds, you would burn 3,500 calories in less time. The reason is that heavier people have to put forth greater effort to do everything. This effect is part of the reason that weight loss slows down after a while. As you lose weight, the number of calories you burn doing a certain activity drops. So to burn the same number of calories—and to lose the same amount of weight—you have to spend more and more time doing it. Table 13-1 gives examples of how people who weigh different amounts burn calories at different speeds.

In Real Life

In reality, you burn calories constantly, even when you are completely still. It takes energy to keep your temperature at 98.6°, digest food, keep your heart beating, and do many, many other tasks. What matters is how many **extra** calories you burn. So you should compare the calories you use during exercise with how many you would burn if you weren't exercising.

A 200-pound person burns about 2 calories a minute resting. So playing the flute, which burns about 3.2 calories per minute, burns only a little more than 1 extra calorie a minute. Although a 200-pound flautist would burn 3,500 calories in less than 19 hours, it would take 48 hours of flute playing to burn 3,500 more calories than just sitting around.

The amount of effort it takes to burn 3,500 more calories than usual is quite a contrast to how little effort it takes to eat 3,500

TABLE 13-1

How Various Activities Burn Calories

ACTIVITY	CALORIES BURNED PER MINUTE FOR A PERSON WHO WEIGHS		
	150 POUNDS	183 POUNDS	216 POUNDS
Sitting quietly	1.4	1.7	2.1
Ironing clothes	2.2	2.7	3.2
Playing the piano	2.7	3.3	3.9
Dancing (ballroom)	3.5	4.2	5.0
Raking	3.7	4.5	5.3
Milking cows by hand	3.7	4.5	5.3
Doing yoga	4.2	5.1	6.1
Vacuuming	4.4	5.4	6.4
Bicycling at 5.5 miles per hour	4.4	5.3	6.3
Washing the car	4.8	5.7	6.9
Walking on a road for fun	5.4	6.6	7.8
Lifting weights	5.8	7.1	8.4
Playing tennis for fun	7.4	9.0	10.7
Water skiing	8.2	10.1	12.0
Riding a motorcycle	9.3	11.3	13.3
Skin-diving	14.0	17.1	20.2

Data based on McArdle WD, Katch FI, Katch VL: *Exercise Physiology.* 4th edition. Baltimore, MD, Williams & Wilkins, 1996, p. 769–781

fewer calories than usual. A medium order of fast-food french fries can be 400 calories or more. If you usually order fries with your lunch and you stop (without ordering something else instead), you will cut 3,500 calories in only 9 days. Depending on the fast-food chain, ordering a hamburger without cheese can save you 50 to 100 calories a day. You'll cut 3,500 calories in 1 to 2 months (if you don't increase the other food you eat).

Put another way, if you weigh 200 pounds, leaving a small slice of cheese off your burger has the same effect on your calorie balance as playing the flute for 42 minutes.

In addition, some scientists believe that the body may change its other activities to make up for the calories you burn exercising. For example, when you've exercised, you may eat more food or be more sedentary the rest of the day to make up for your activity. If so, that would reduce the benefit of exercise.

There are other reasons why exercise doesn't work as well as cutting calories to help people lose weight.

First, people who are overweight are often in poor shape and can't exercise long enough to burn more than a small number of extra calories. Cutting back on food intake doesn't take physical strength or stamina.

Second, some people just don't enjoy exercise. A person who enjoys eating still has that pleasure on a reduced-calorie diet. But a person who enjoys quiet pursuits needs to give up some of that quiet to add exercise. Getting yourself to do things you don't enjoy over and over again is very hard.

Scientists have many different views on exercise and weight. Some believe that exercise suppresses appetite, so people may eat fewer calories on the days they exercise. (Of course, as you learned a few paragraphs ago, other scientists think exercising increases how much people eat later in the day.) Some scientists believe that exercise changes people's taste preferences so that they eat less fat. Some believe that the improvements exercise makes to mood and self-esteem help people stick to their new habits. And some believe that exercise may increase the body's calorie burning. Any of these factors, if true, would boost the benefit of exercise.

THE IMPORTANCE OF BEING REGULAR

Whether you are exercising for health, for fitness, for strength, for good glucose control, or for weight loss, regularity is important. The effects of exercise disappear quickly. If you stop, your glucose level will go back up, and your muscles will lose their tone.

About half of people who start exercising stop before 6 months have passed. Chapters 20 and 21 will discuss ways to keep up good habits once you start. In the meantime, keeping these principles in mind will help:

- Choose activities that are fun.

- Start slowly and work up to longer and more vigorous activities.

- Don't expect to become fit or thin right away. It takes awhile for the effects of exercise to show.

- Don't get mad at yourself for lapses. Ignore them and pick up where you left off.

OLDER PEOPLE AND EXERCISE

In general, age is no reason not to exercise. In fact, exercise is usually quite good for older people. Many of the problems people think of as caused by getting older are often instead caused by not being active enough.

If you have started having trouble with your daily activities, exercise can help. Aerobic exercise will give you more endurance. It will then be easier to do housework and yard chores. Strengthening exercise can build up weak, unstable muscles. It will then be easier to open windows, get up from chairs, and climb stairs. Stretching can make you more flexible. It will then be easier to get dressed and get in the bathtub. Because of these benefits, older people who exercise stay independent longer—as much as 10 to 20 years longer.

The older you are, the more time you've had to accumulate injuries and diseases. So it's extra important for older people to talk to their doctors before starting to exercise. Exercise is a good treatment for many diseases, such as high blood pressure, arthritis, and heart disease. Talking to your doctor first will help you design an exercise program that will improve your physical condition without worsening illnesses and injuries you already have.

When doing aerobic exercises, older people generally do best if they exercise less intensely and for shorter time—but more often—than younger people. For example, older people might exercise 5 to 10 minutes at a time rather than the 15 to 60 minutes a young person does. The length that's best to exercise depends on how fit you are and will increase as you progress.

Older people tend to have less water in their bodies. So drinking water before, during, and after exercising is even more important. Because older joints are less cushioned, high-impact exercises (such as running) may be painful.

Just like young people, older people should choose exercises they enjoy. The most popular activities for Americans over 65 are walking and gardening. But there's no reason not to choose a more lively sport, such as cross-country skiing or tennis, if your doctor okays it.

EVERYONE IS DIFFERENT

Some people are born more active than others. Some people have more athletic talent than others.

Scientists' current views about exercise are particularly good news for people who enjoy thinking, sewing, or painting more than running, playing basketball, or climbing Mount Everest. People who find peace and joy in stillness don't have to take up a vigorous hobby they hate to improve their health. Rather, they can sneak in their 30 minutes of activity each day around things they have to do anyway (vacuuming the house, cleaning the garage) or things they enjoy (walking to the fabric shop or the bookstore, scouting out scenic locations to paint).

The Skinny on Chapter

13

▶ You can improve your health by being moderately active for 30 minutes or more a day, 5 days or more per week.

▶ You don't need to participate in sports or be an athlete to improve your health. Commonplace activities such as washing the car, gardening, raking leaves, or dancing count.

▶ Moderate exercise can be defined as exercise that gets your heart beating at roughly 50% to 70% of its maximum rate or as exercise that allows you to hold a conversation.

▶ You can meet your 30-minute-per-day goal by doing 10 minutes here and 10 minutes there.

▶ You can get even more benefits from exercise by increasing how hard, how long, or how much you exercise.

▶ People with type 2 diabetes can improve their glucose levels by exercising regularly.

▶ Exercising often doesn't help people lose weight, but it does seem to help people keep from gaining or regaining weight.

5

If You Have a Lot of Weight to Lose, Modern Medicine Has Some Extra Help to Offer.

Adopting a lifestyle of restrained eating is the best way for many people to lose weight. But sometimes, it is not enough. When overweight is really hurting your health, you may need a more aggressive strategy. This section will tell you about three options for losing weight with the help of your doctor. Very-low-calorie diets produce quick, large weight loss. Drugs can help people lose more weight. Surgery is a drastic measure that can sometimes save lives.

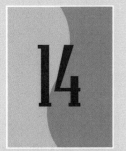

14

Eating a very
restricted diet for just
a few months can
jump-start your
weight-loss effort.

Very-Low-Calorie Diets

I f you look hard enough, you can find an exception to most rules.

This chapter is one of those exceptions.

This book stresses that short-term lifestyle changes produce only short-term results. To lose weight for good, people need to adopt new habits and keep them up for the rest of their lives.

Yet here, only halfway through the book, is an exception to that rule: very-low-calorie diets. When a meal plan provides 800 or fewer calories per day, it's called a very-low-calorie diet. Clearly, no one can eat a diet this low in energy for long. So a very-low-calorie diet is not a permanent answer to a weight problem. On the other hand, as this chapter will show, a very-low-calorie diet can be a good way to start a weight-loss effort.

WHAT A VERY-LOW-CALORIE DIET IS— AND ISN'T

Because eating so few calories carries some risk, some definitions are in order.

A very-low-calorie diet is:

- Supervised by a doctor—perhaps your own doctor, a doctor who specializes in obesity, or a doctor at a reputable weight-loss clinic

- High in protein so that lean tissues such as muscles don't waste away

- Fortified with vitamins and minerals

- Based either on drinking a powder that you mix with a liquid or on eating very lean meat

- Suitable for people who are truly overweight and at high risk for health problems, but not for people who just want to lose 10 pounds

- Not suitable to try by yourself

- Not the same as the liquid-protein diets that killed people in the 1970s

- Not the same as powders sold in drugstores and supermarkets for losing weight

HOW WELL THEY WORK

Very-low-calorie diets take weight off well. Over the 3 to 4 months that a very-low-calorie diet might last, people can lose 40 pounds. This is at least double the weight loss produced by a standard reduced-calorie food plan. In studies of very-low-calorie diets, 9 of 10 people lose at least 22 pounds. On standard low-calorie food plans, only 6 of 10 people lose this much weight.

One reason that very-low-calorie diets may take off so many pounds is that they are based on controlled portion sizes. Usually, a person buys a liquid diet. It's hard to eat too much by accident when you have a quota of liquid diet assigned for each day. In contrast, when people eat real food, it's hard to keep track of every single bite every single day. Several studies have shown that people often misjudge how much they eat. People on commercially prepared very-low-calorie diets do not need to worry about these problems.

Another reason very-low-calorie diets work may be that they suppress hunger. After the first few days, many people say they no longer feel hungry.

After the very-low-calorie diet is over, people start to gain back the weight they lost. Most regain all the weight within 5 years. Just as with every other weight-loss plan, people who go on very-low-calorie diets need to make changes in their daily habits if they want to keep the weight off. (See the box "Spotlight on Research: A Commercial Very-Low-Calorie Program.")

SPOTLIGHT ON RESEARCH
A Commercial Very-Low-Calorie Program

Research shows that very-low-calorie diets can help people lose a lot of weight. But, just as with standard reduced-calorie eating plans, weight comes back easily. These conclusions were supported in a 1997 *International Journal of Eating Disorders* article. This reported the results of yearly surveys of 621 people who had completed a very-low-calorie diet program in 1989. (The formula's manufacturer sponsored the survey.) By the end of a 26-week treatment program, the women had lost an average of 52 pounds (about 23% of their weight). Men had lost an average of 75 pounds (about 26% of their weight).

Two years after the treatment program, when researchers first surveyed these people, they found that women had regained an average of 31 pounds and men, an average of 37. Weight regain slowed as time went by. By the end of the fifth year, almost half the sample had dropped out of the study for one reason or another. The remaining women had kept off 12 of the 52 pounds they had lost, and men had kept off 23 of the 75 pounds they had lost.

Because a 5% weight loss is thought to provide health benefits, the researchers looked to see how many of the remaining subjects kept off at least this much weight after 5 years. Twenty-eight percent of women and 58% of men had met this definition of success. People varied greatly, though, in how much weight came back. At the final survey, about one in nine was at least 20% below his or her starting weight. On the other hand, 15% of women and 9% of men weighed more than they had before they joined the program.

Clearly, adopting a plan for long-term calorie restraint is necessary to stay at a lower weight, no matter how you lose it in the first place.

Risks and Cautions

You should weigh the risks and benefits of very-low-calorie diets just as you would those of any other medical procedure. Here are a few things to think about.

It can be hard to get enough protein, vitamins, and minerals when so few calories are eaten.

Any time someone loses a lot of weight fairly quickly, the risk of gallstones shoots up. Studies have found that one-tenth to one-quarter of people who go on very-low-calorie diets get gallstones. Hair may also fall out, and some people feel tired.

Researchers suspect that food deprivation may cause some people to become binge eaters. (See "Talking About Binge Eating.")

Because of these various side effects, a doctor experienced in very-low-calorie diets should always oversee one. Depending on the plan, you may also need to buy a formula. As a result, very-low-calorie diets can be a costly way to lose weight. Whether you work with one of your own doctors or go to a commercial weight-loss program, be sure to ask at the start about the expected costs of checkups, liquid diets, and supplements.

TALKING ABOUT BINGE EATING

What is binge eating?

Binge eating means a person has episodes in which he or she eats large amounts of food in a brief time without being able to stop. Another name for binge eating is compulsive overeating. Men make up one-fourth to one-third of binge eaters.

What is the link between eating restrictions and binge eating?

Some researchers believe that dieting—temporarily adopting stringent eating habits to lose weight—may predispose people to eating

TALKING ABOUT BINGE EATING *Continued*

disorders. Some studies have found that most people who binge start doing so while on a diet. Whatever mental effects dieting has, they're not the same in everyone. Most American women diet. But most never get an eating disorder. It's not just purposeful dieting that is linked to bingeing. For example, some prisoners of war who've had too little to eat binge after release.

It's unclear whether bingeing is caused by the actual physical deprivation, by psychological deprivation, or by the stress of not being able to eat what one wants.

What about very-low-calorie diets?
Do scientific studies link them to binge eating?

Only a handful of studies have looked specifically at very-low-calorie diets and bingeing. Their results are inconsistent.

The longest of these studies was reported in the *International Journal of Obesity* in 1996. Finnish researchers followed 62 overweight adults between 20 and 60 years old who went on a very-low-calorie diet. They used three questionnaires to measure binge eating before and several times after the diet. Right after the diet, the subjects had the fewest symptoms of binge eating. Over the next 2 years, binge-eating symptoms gradually returned. In people who regained weight, binge-eating symptoms returned to pre-diet levels. But people who were able to maintain their weight loss had only small increases in binge-eating symptoms.

In this study, a very-low-calorie diet did not increase binge eating. In fact, it decreased bingeing for a while. But people whose bingeing symptoms came back were not able to maintain their weight loss.

More studies are needed to tease apart the causes and effects of binge eating.

The last problem with very-low-calorie diets is one you already know about. Weight loss is brief unless people make changes in their life. One of the most vital of these is not to let calorie intake creep up over time, but to keep it level.

VERY-LOW-CALORIE DIETS AND DIABETES

Very-low-calorie diets are not suitable for people with type 1 diabetes because they may cause low-blood-glucose reactions. People who have kidney disease also should not use them because only healthy kidneys can process a high-protein diet.

Very-low-calorie diets do seem to work well for people with type 2 diabetes with healthy kidneys. Glucose levels fall within a few days, and most people can stop taking their diabetes drugs. (See the box "Spotlight on Research: Off-and-On Diets.")

WHO SHOULD USE THEM

The American Obesity Association (a group that promotes obesity research and care) and Shape Up America! (a group that promotes better fitness) issued guidelines in 1996 to help doctors help people lose weight. These guidelines say that very-low-calorie diets are suitable for people whose weight puts them at high risk of other health problems. They define a "high risk" for a person with diabetes as a body mass index (see Chapter 1) higher than 27.

These guidelines say that pregnant women, people with unstable medical or mental conditions, people who have diseases that are going to kill them, and people with eating disorders should not start any weight-loss program. The guidelines warn that doctors should be careful about putting certain people, including those with type 1 diabetes, on a very-low-calorie diet.

SPOTLIGHT ON RESEARCH
Off-and-On Diets

Because of the good effect of very-low-calorie diets on glucose levels, some researchers have studied whether going on and off very-low-calorie diets might be worthwhile. University of Pittsburgh researchers have studied off-and-on diets without finding much benefit. For example, in results published in the *American Journal of Medicine* in 1994, the researchers compared two diets in adults with type 2 diabetes. For one group, the goal was to eat 1,000 to 1,200 calories per day.

People in the other group first spent 12 weeks on a very-low-calorie diet of 500 calories a day. They then spent 12 weeks working up to and then eating a 1,000- to 1,200-calorie diet. They then repeated this cycle. Both groups also went to weekly behavioral therapy sessions for a year.

Both groups lost weight for the first 6 months, then started regaining. After 1 year, the off-and-on diet group had lost somewhat more weight (an average of 31 pounds vs. 23 pounds for those on the low-calorie diet). But almost all of the weight loss occurred during the first 12 weeks on the very-low-calorie diet. In both groups, the people who had lost the most weight regained the most. So after 2 years, the amount of weight loss was roughly equal. After 1 year, both groups had improved their diabetes control about equally, although fewer people in the very-low-calorie group needed diabetes drugs.

This study shows that very-low-calorie diets work about as well for people with diabetes as they do for other people. They increase weight loss. Weight regain is still a problem, just as with other weight-loss plans. But there seems to be little benefit to cycling on and off a very-low-calorie diet.

The Skinny on Chapter

14

► When a weight-loss plan is based on eating fewer than 800 calories per day, it is called a very-low-calorie diet.

► Because a very-low-calorie diet is a form of starvation, people stay on it for only a few months.

► Very-low-calorie diets often consist of a high-protein, vitamin-fortified drink.

► Weight loss on a very-low-calorie diet is often double that on a standard low-calorie eating plan.

► Any very-low-calorie diet, including those offered by commercial weight-loss clinics, should be supervised by a doctor.

► Very-low-calorie diets can be costly.

► After the diet is over, pounds tend to come back.

► As with any other form of weight loss, only changes in habits, including long-term calorie restraint, keep pounds off.

► Overweight people with type 2 diabetes who have healthy kidneys are often suitable candidates for very-low-calorie diets. People with type 1 diabetes are not.

► Very-low-calorie diets have good effects on blood glucose levels in people with type 2 diabetes.

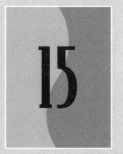
Appetite-Suppressant Drugs

Appetite suppressants turn off hunger in some people. Used with caution, such drugs can help some people lose weight when attempts to cut calories are not successful by themselves.

Who hasn't wished for a magic pill at some point in life—perhaps a pill that would clear up pimples or build big muscles or cause fat to melt away? Unfortunately, medicine rarely lives up to people's fantasies of an easy, safe fix for problems.

Weight-loss pills are no exception. As you've already seen, your health is likely to improve if you take off some excess pounds. You may be tempted by what seems an easy route to weight loss—a weight-loss pill.

In fact, weight-loss drugs are not magic. No weight-loss pill takes off excess fat by itself. Rather, weight-loss drugs work only if you cut calorie intake (by eating less food) and increase calorie burning (by being more active). Like any other drug, weight-loss drugs have side effects and can interact with other drugs. So you should talk to your doctor before you use any of them.

This chapter will introduce you to the various weight-loss drugs now on the market and tell you how they work and about their side effects.

This chapter will also provide a quickie look at the ways drugs of the future might help the body lose weight.

TRAITS OF WEIGHT-LOSS DRUGS

The drugs currently approved for weight loss act by dampening appetite, by affecting fat absorption, or by increasing a sense of fullness. If people are less hungry, they should find it easier to stick to a reduced-calorie diet.

But hunger is not the only reason people eat. If someone on a weight-loss drug continues to eat as much food as before, he or she will lose no weight. So weight-loss pills are used **with** a reduced-calorie diet and increased physical activity, not instead of them.

In general, people who take weight-loss drugs lose an extra 4 to 40 pounds (although, as with any drug, people vary in how well they respond—some lose more than 100 pounds). Drugs help people lose weight for about 6 months, and after that, no more pounds are usually lost. But some people do continue to lose weight.

Studies of weight-loss drugs that lasted more than 6 months are few. But these longer studies do show that the drugs don't stop working after 6 months. Rather, the drugs' action then is to maintain weight loss by slowing or stopping regain.

Obesity is a chronic condition, just like high blood pressure. If people get good results from a blood pressure drug, they don't expect the effect to last after they stop taking the drug. So it is with weight-loss drugs. If the drug is stopped, it stops working. Unless a person continues to restrict calories, the weight comes back.

Weight-Loss Drugs That Act on Brain Chemicals

Drugs That Affect Catecholamines. The catecholamines are brain chemicals that make people feel less hungry.

Four current prescription drugs are in this class. Three of these drugs boost the production of catecholamines. These are diethylpropion, phentermine, and phendimetrazine. A fourth drug, mazindol, acts instead by keeping nerves from removing catecholamines from the gaps between the nerves. All four have been used for many years and have similar side effects (see Table 15-1). They are controlled substances, but are not addictive.

TABLE 15-1

Modern Prescription Drugs for Weight Loss

GENERIC NAME AND SOME BRAND NAMES	SOME POSSIBLE SIDE EFFECTS	MAY NOT BE SUITABLE FOR PEOPLE WHO:*
Diethylpropion (Tenuate, Tenuate Dospan, Tepanil, M-Orexic)	Insomnia, jitteriness, increased blood pressure	■ Take MAO inhibitors ■ Have severe heart disease, hyperthyroidism, high blood pressure, hardening of the arteries, or epilepsy ■ Have a history of substance abuse
Mazindol (Mazanor, Sanorex)	Dry mouth, constipation, insomnia, jitteriness, increased heart rate	■ Take MAO inhibitors ■ Have glaucoma ■ Have a history of substance abuse
Phendimetrazine (Adipost, Anorex, Bontril, Plegine, Prelu-2, X-Trozine, and many others)	Insomnia, jitteriness, increased heart rate	■ Take MAO inhibitors or stimulants ■ Have hyperthyroidism, high blood pressure, heart disease, glaucoma, or hardening of the arteries ■ Have a history of substance abuse
Phentermine (Adipex-P, Fastin, Ionamin, and many others)	Insomnia, jitteriness, increased heart rate	■ Take MAO inhibitors ■ Have hyperthyroidism, high blood pressure, heart disease, glaucoma, or hardening of the arteries ■ Have a history of substance abuse
Sibutramine (Meridia)	Constipation, dry mouth, insomnia, increased blood pressure	■ Take MAO inhibitors ■ Have heart disease (including irregular heartbeats) or uncontrolled or poorly controlled high blood pressure ■ Have had a stroke ■ Have kidney disease, liver disease, or glaucoma
Orlistat (Xenical)	Oily, liquid, or loose stools, abdominal pain, gas	■ To be determined

*Most weight-loss drugs are not suitable for children or pregnant women. Also, you should tell your doctor if you have ever had an allergic reaction to an appetite suppressant or an amphetamine. As when getting any new drug, always tell your doctor what other prescription and over-the-counter drugs and herbs you are taking. Also make sure your doctor knows about your diabetes and any eating disorders or other medical conditions you have.

Phenylpropanolamine is a related appetite suppressant and is the only effective weight-loss drug you can buy without a prescription. (It is also used in many decongestants to stop runny noses.) Don't use an excessive dose because it could increase your blood pressure. Side effects of phenylpropanolamine include dry mouth and insomnia.

The earliest drugs in this class that were used to help people lose weight were the amphetamines. Doctors generally believe they should not be prescribed because they are quite addictive. They also have so many side effects and dangers that taking them is much riskier than being overweight.

Drugs That Increase Serotonin Release. Serotonin is a brain chemical that plays roles in both mood and appetite. When serotonin levels are high, people feel full longer. So they are inclined to eat less.

Some drugs that used to be available acted by causing more serotonin to be released. They were withdrawn because of serious potential side effects. One of these, fenfluramine (Pondimin), had been around for a long time. It was approved by the FDA in 1973 and was withdrawn in 1997. The other, dexfenfluramine (brand name Redux), contained the same active ingredient and was approved by the FDA in 1996 and withdrawn in 1997. Both were very popular and used by millions of people. (They were sometimes used in combination with another weight-loss drug mentioned above, phentermine, and that drug is still available.)

The manufacturers withdrew the two fenfluramine drugs from the market when they were linked to increased rates of two serious conditions, primary pulmonary hypertension, or PPH, and an unusual heart valve disorder. PPH is a serious disease of the arteries of the lungs. Its symptoms include shortness of breath, chest pain, faintness, and swelling in the lower legs and ankles. (If you've taken any weight-loss drug and have these symptoms, see your doctor. PPH has been linked to use of weight-loss drugs other than dexfenfluramine and fenfluramine, although the evidence is weaker.) Valvular heart disease involves an unusual thickening of the valve so it can't open and close as it should.

Although links between a drug and a disease do not prove that the drug causes the disease, and the effects may be different in different people, the concerns about the seriousness of these potential side effects are merited. If you have used either of these drugs, the manufacturers and the United States government recommend that you talk with your doctor. (See the box "What Should People Who Took Fenfluramine or Dexfenfluramine Do?".)

WHAT SHOULD PEOPLE WHO TOOK FENFLURAMINE OR DEXFENFLURAMINE DO?

Millions of Americans took dexfenfluramine (Redux) or fenfluramine (Pondimin, part of the popular phen/fen combination) before these drugs were removed from the U.S. market. They were withdrawn in September 1997 because their use was linked both to a lung disease called primary pulmonary hypertension and to a heart valve disorder.

On November 13, 1997, the Department of Health and Human Services released interim (temporary) recommendations for people who took either drug. The recommendations say that these people should do three things:

First, see a doctor. The doctor should take a complete medical history and examine you for evidence of heart or lung disease.

Second, if the doctor finds signs that you might have heart or lung disease, you should have an echocardiogram. (An echocardiogram is an ultrasound of the heart. Sound waves are bounced off the heart—a painless procedure—to create an image of the heart as it beats.)

Third, if the doctor finds no sign that you have heart or lung disease, you should still have an echocardiogram to look for valve problems in one situation: If you are to have certain dental or medical procedures that can allow bacteria into the bloodstream.

It is important for people who have a valve disorder to find out about it. People with leaky heart valves should take antibiotics before procedures that can let bacteria enter the bloodstream. The reason is that these people are prone to getting bacteria infections of the lining of the heart and the covering of the valves. This infection is called "bacterial endocarditis."

The American Heart Association (AHA) issued guidelines in June 1997 for antibiotic use. (To find out how to contact the AHA, see the RESOURCES section of this book.) In general, antibiotics are recommended before procedures involving the gastrointestinal tract

Continued

WHAT SHOULD PEOPLE WHO TOOK FENFLURAMINE OR DEXFENFLURAMINE DO? *Continued*

and the urinary tract—that is, the systems that process food and drink from the time you ingest them until what's left leaves the body as waste. According to the AHA guidelines, people with valve disease should take antibiotics before tooth cleaning, tooth removal, gum surgery, and removal of the tonsils, among other procedures.

To be on the safe side, if you have a valve problem, always talk to your doctor before having any dental work or medical procedure. Your doctor can then write you a prescription if antibiotics are advisable.

One more complication was seen when animals were given very large amounts of dexfenfluramine or fenfluramine. They caused long-lasting drops in serotonin levels in the brain, suggesting that some brain cells might be damaged. These changes might not happen in people, but only more research can tell us that.

Herbal phen/fen products have been marketed as natural alternatives to the prescription drugs phentermine and fenfluramine. The FDA considers these products to be unapproved drugs. It warns that they have not been shown to be safe or effective and may contain ingredients that have been associated with health risks. Despite their advertising, these products do not contain fenfluramine.

Drugs That Act to Slow the Inactivation of Brain Chemicals. Boosting the release of brain chemicals is not the only way a drug can increase their concentrations. Some drugs slow the inactivation of brain chemicals such as norepinephrine, serotonin, and dopamine. Because these chemicals continue to be active longer, they continue to exert their effects on the brain longer. One such effect can be on appetite.

One new drug in this class is sibutramine (brand name Meridia), which was approved for weight loss and maintenance in 1997. This drug may help to counter the tendency to overeat by enhancing the feeling of fullness. Similar drugs such as fluoxetine (Prozac) are best for depression and have not been approved to treat obesity.

One possible side effect of sibutramine is increased blood pressure and heart rate. In studies of this drug, some people showed big increases. Most, however, had only small increases and did not have to stop taking the drug. If you are taking this drug, you should have your blood pressure checked regularly.

Weight-Loss Drugs That Affect the Absorption of Food From the Intestines

A new class of weight-loss drug affects how your body absorbs food. This kind of drug does not reduce appetite much, but rather reduces the calories the body gets to use. It does so by keeping some of the enzymes in the stomach and intestines from doing their jobs.

The first new drug in this class is orlistat (brand name Xenical). An FDA advisory committee recommended in 1997 that orlistat be approved.

Orlistat helps with both weight loss and prevention of weight regain. It works by inhibiting lipase. That is, it interferes with enzymes that help the body absorb fat from food. Orlistat keeps the body from absorbing about 30% of the fat it takes in.

SPOTLIGHT ON RESEARCH
Sibutramine and Valvular Heart Disease

Two studies reported in the package insert for the drug sibutramine aimed to make sure that there was no link between sibutramine and heart valve disorder.

In one study, 210 patients received sibutramine (15 mg) or a placebo (fake pill). Echocardiograms showed no difference in the number of patients who had valvular heart disease between the two groups. In another study, 25 patients were examined before and after treatment with sibutramine. There were no cases of valvular heart disease.

Of course, researchers will continue to study sibutramine for any possible risks.

Of course, the fat that gets eaten but doesn't get absorbed has to go someplace. It goes through the intestinal tract and can cause lots of usually minor side effects. The most common side effects, oily or loose stools and gas, usually go away after awhile. Because the drug may interfere with absorption of vitamins as well as fat, it's probably a good idea to be sure you get enough vitamins.

You may already be familiar with another drug that interferes with absorption, acarbose (Precose), which is approved to help people with diabetes slow the absorption of complex carbohydrates. This drug can reduce peak levels of glucose after a meal, but it doesn't appear to be useful for weight loss.

In the future, we may find that certain combinations of different drugs work best together. But for now, it's best not to combine weight-loss drugs until their effects together have been well studied.

THINKING ABOUT WEIGHT-LOSS DRUGS AND THEIR SAFETY

Two issues of great concern to doctors and patients alike are how long people should take weight-loss drugs and how likely they are to help someone.

Short-Term or Long-Term Use? Beliefs about weight-loss drugs have long intertwined with beliefs about obese people. Once, not so long ago, doctors viewed being overweight as a personality flaw and losing weight as a matter of willpower. Doctors assumed that if people would just show some self-control for a change, they would be cured. For this reason, weight-loss drugs were tested only for brief times—often less than 6 months. When weight came back after the drugs were stopped, they were thought to be failures.

Of course, by these standards, every treatment for overweight is a failure. Cutting calories stops working when you go back to old eating habits. Exercise no longer helps once you stop. The reason, scientists now know, is that obesity is not a short-term problem. No short-term effort keeps pounds off. Weight only stays off if people adopt new habits forever.

It's now obvious that weight-loss drugs would probably work best if taken forever. So the short-term trials of the past are not good enough now. Since 1995, the FDA has required companies seeking approval of new weight-loss drugs to test them long term. Phentermine, mazindol, and sibutramine have been studied for at least 1 year.

Can Drugs Help Everyone? You may have noticed that summaries of studies in this book tend to list only results for the average person. But averages don't give the whole picture. For example, there are many ways the average weight loss in a study of 10 people can be 10 pounds. Three very different ones are:

- Everyone lost 10 pounds.

- One person lost 100 pounds, and no one else lost weight.

- Five people each lost 20 pounds, and the others lost no weight.

Some studies of weight-loss drugs have looked at these individual differences. As a result, we know that people have a wide range of responses. Some people lose no weight at all. Some people lose a good deal of weight. And some lose a little. Doctors also have found that people may respond well to one weight-loss drug, but not respond to another. Usually you can tell within 4 to 6 weeks whether a drug is helping. If it's not, you and your doctor need to talk about changing the dose or stopping the drug.

Safety. Although most side effects of currently available drugs are mild, clearly we don't yet know every possible problem. Sometimes, drugs are linked to problems that are either hard to measure or are very rare and so are hard to identify—for example, the concerns that got dexfenfluramine and fenfluramine removed from the market.

WHO SHOULD CONSIDER WEIGHT-LOSS DRUGS?

Several organizations have issued guidelines to help doctors prescribe weight-loss drugs.

The guidelines of the American Obesity Association and Shape Up America! were issued in 1996. These guidelines suggest that doctors consider weight-loss drugs only for people whose weight puts them at high risk of other health problems. According to these guidelines, "high risk" for a person with diabetes is a body mass index (BMI; see Chapter 1) greater than 27.

These guidelines say that people who are pregnant or who have unstable medical or mental conditions, fatal diseases, or eating disorders should not enter any weight-loss program. The guidelines also warn that doctors should not put women who are breastfeeding on weight-loss drugs. (Doctors also interpret this caution to apply to women who are trying to become pregnant.)

In 1996, the National Task Force on the Prevention and Treatment of Obesity also issued guidelines for the long-term use of weight-loss drugs. It said that such drugs should not be used routinely in obese people, but may help certain ones, such as those who have obesity-related diseases or who have tried and failed to lose weight by other methods.

The North American Association for the Study of Obesity is a group of scientists who do research to help the obese and to find the causes of obesity. Its 1995 guidelines suggest limiting drugs for people without other conditions to those with a BMI of at least 27. They also say that drug therapy is suitable for obese people with diabetes or other weight-related conditions, but they do not suggest a cutoff BMI for them.

The American Society of Bariatric Physicians also issued guidelines. These say that weight-loss drugs may be appropriate when a person with no other health conditions has a BMI of at least 27 or when a woman is more than 30% fat or a man is more than 25% fat.

One common thread in these guidelines and others is that weight-loss drugs should never be used merely to look better. They should be used only to lower the health risks of excess weight.

DRUGS OF THE FUTURE

Scientists are working on many new drugs to treat overweight. Over the next few years, several of these may come on the market.

Drugs Based on Hunger-Control Peptides

One way your brain knows what you've eaten is that your stomach and intestines release many small proteins (peptides). Some of these so-called gut peptides signal to the brain that you need to eat. Some tell your brain you've had enough. Doctors are now testing whether blocking or enhancing these peptides could aid in weight loss.

TALKING ABOUT DRUGS IN THE NEWS

I'm always hearing about new obesity genes being discovered or new diabetes treatments. But then nothing happens. Why?

It's a long way from the lab bench to your drugstore's shelves. Pretend that today, someone discovers a protein that might cure overweight. Scientists would test it in animals to make sure it slims them down without making them sick. If it does, then scientists would test it in humans to see if it were safe to take. If so, it would be tested to see what doses work best. After that, still more tests would be performed. These layers of trials take years. If the drug makes it that far, it still has to jump another high hurdle—approval by the FDA. The FDA takes more than a year to review the mountain of data on each proposed drug and its proposed labeling. Even if the FDA approves the drug, it may not go on sale at once. The company needs to make enough drug to fill the orders.

How can I separate the truth from the hype?

- Be wary of claims that a newly discovered compound is a sure cure or could be available within a couple of years. It takes an average of 8 1/2 years from the start of human trials to FDA approval—and that's only after animal trials are done and only if the trials have good results.

- Watch out for words like "breakthrough," "first," "most important," "revolutionary," and "cure." They're usually not true.

- Keep in mind that enthusiasm is sometimes misplaced.

- Ask your doctor or diabetes educator about discoveries that sound promising. If the drug or gene really is important, he or she will have heard of it and can fill you in on what the news stories left out.

- Learn more about diabetes and your weight. Your best protection against being taken in is to know enough about diabetes to recognize mistakes and half-truths.

Neuropeptide Y. Neuropeptide Y (NPY) increases hunger for carbo-hydrates. It may also reduce how much fat people burn. Several companies are testing drugs that would block NPY's action.

Cholecystokinin. Cholecystokinin, or CCK, decreases appetite for all kinds of food. It slows the emptying of the stomach. Two kinds of drugs under development affect CCK. One kind makes the body respond better to CCK. The other kind keeps CCK from being broken down in the body, which slows the return of hunger.

Galanin. Galanin is a peptide that increases hunger for both fat and carbohydrate. Researchers are exploring whether blocking the action of galanin could lead to weight loss.

Drugs That Burn Calories

It's possible that some drugs could kick the body's energy-burning into high gear. In fact, some scientists believe that current weight-loss drugs may work in part by increasing energy use.

Beta-Adrenergic Agonists. Drugs called beta-adrenergic agonists make mice and rats burn fat even though they eat the same amount of food as usual. These drugs also greatly improve glucose control in rats and mice with experimental diabetes. Several companies are working to develop beta-adrenergic agonists that do the same things in humans.

Drugs That Mimic Hormones

Some possible drugs are wholly or partly copies of hormones and other body proteins that carry messages (such as the gut peptides). These copies of proteins are called "mimics."

CCK Mimic. One drug company is testing a drug that would act just as CCK does in the body. The drug would slow the emptying of the stomach and tell the body to stop eating.

Dopamine Mimics. Dopamine is a brain chemical with many roles in the body. Bromocriptine is a dopamine mimic that is already used in the United States to treat Parkinson's disease and diverse other conditions. Researchers are testing whether it can also lower blood glucose in people with diabetes. It may be tested for helping people lose weight as well.

A GIFT FOR HIS CHILDREN

"**I** was just waiting for my heart attack," says Roger Esfahani, describing his life before weight-loss drugs. Esfahani has had severe thyroid and pituitary problems since childhood. These conditions stunted his growth while increasing his girth. "In college, I grew up to almost 400 pounds. I was diagnosed [type 2] diabetic when I was 19 in 1977, at the height of my weight," says Esfahani. Treatment of his diabetes eventually helped him to lose more than 100 pounds.

But life as a prosecutor is stressful, and Esfahani began gaining weight. By September 1995, he hit 323 pounds and was taking 224 units of Regular insulin and 90 units of ultralente insulin a day. "My doctor and I sat down and we talked about it. He said we need to do something very drastic, and I agreed," says Esfahani. He started taking a combination of fenfluramine and phentermine.

The results were rapid. "I started taking it on a Friday night, and by Sunday night I had my first terrible low [glucose reaction]," says Esfahani. He needed to cut his insulin dose the very first week because his glucose levels kept falling too low. In 3 months, he lost 28 pounds, and his diabetes control improved drastically, even though he was down to 122 units of Regular and 82 units of ultralente a day. In addition, he began sleeping better, his HDL (good) cholesterol level went up, and the pain from diabetic nerve damage in his feet eased.

"The side effects are minimal," he says. "I had dry mouth for about 6 weeks or so. I developed acne on my scalp and torso." Esfahani knows that even after he reaches his target weight of 230, he probably will stay on drug treatment the rest of his life to keep from regaining the weight. But he says it's worth it to be able to watch his children grow up.

Urocortin Mimic. People who are stressed often lose their appetite. The peptide responsible may be urocortin. One company is working on a urocortin mimic that would make hunger disappear.

Drugs Based on Genes

Genes are a set of coded instructions for building proteins. The set of all the instructions together is enough to construct a complete person. Sometimes a mutation (mistake) in a gene causes it to make a defective protein or not produce one at all. A disease may then result.

The discovery of genes that underlie obesity or diabetes in humans could lead to exciting new treatments. Once scientists know what causes a medical problem, possible ways to fix it sometimes seem obvious. For example, if a disease is caused by too much of a certain protein, scientists might try to stop its production or block it from acting. If the body is ill because it lacks a protein, scientists might try to prod the body into making more or might provide it in pills or shots.

Scientists have found many gene mutations that can cause obesity in mice and rats. But so far, they have found only two gene mutations that cause obesity in humans. These two mutations are very, very rare. Probably in people, many different genes contribute at the same time to cause obesity, and these genes are probably influenced by the environment. As of now, more than 75 genes or markers for genes have been identified as possibly involved in human obesity.

The weight-related proteins attracting the lion's share of interest among scientists today are leptin and the uncoupling proteins.

Leptin. In mice, leptin is the protein that tells the brain when the body contains enough fat. Mice that lack leptin become very fat and get type 2 diabetes. So far, only two obese people have been found who lack leptin. Even so, many scientists are studying leptin, and one company is testing it as a weight-loss drug in humans.

Uncoupling Proteins. The uncoupling proteins appear to control energy use in cells. Differences among people in uncoupling proteins may underlie differences in metabolic rate (how fast people burn energy). One of the uncoupling proteins may even be the "thrifty gene" (see Chapter 1).

The Skinny on Chapter

▸ Weight-loss drugs can boost weight loss in people who are also cutting calories.

▸ Like any other drugs, weight-loss drugs have risks and side effects.

▸ Current weight-loss drugs help people lose weight by making them less hungry and helping them take in fewer calories.

▸ Because obesity is a long-term problem, scientists believe that treatments must be long-term as well. But the safety of weight-loss drugs when used for many years is unknown.

▸ Drugs that reduce appetite by working on brain chemicals called catecholamines are diethylpropion, phentermine, phendimetrazine, mazindol, and phenylpropanolamine.

▸ A drug that acts to slow the inactivation of appetite-related brain chemicals is sibutramine.

▸ In contrast, orlistat does not act on brain chemicals. Instead, it reduces the absorption of fat from the intestines.

▸ Because of the known side effects of weight-loss drugs and the unknown long-term effects, scientists agree they are suitable only for people at high risk of weight-related health problems.

▸ Choosing a reputable doctor is important if you are thinking about using weight-loss drugs.

▸ Some future drugs may boost or suppress peptides that keep the brain informed about whether the body needs to eat.

▸ Some future drugs may make the body burn more calories.

▸ Some future drugs may act in the body just like natural hormones or peptides.

▸ Genes are a set of instructions that tell cells how to make proteins.

▸ Gene mutations (mistakes) can cause obesity in mice and rats, and there are probably many genes involved in causing obesity in humans.

▸ Scientists are studying many proteins that may be related to weight. Some are leptin and the uncoupling proteins.

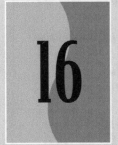

16

For people with
severe obesity,
stomach surgery may
provide long-term
weight control.

Surgery for Weight Loss

"For extreme illnesses, extreme treatments are most fitting," the great physician Hippocrates said. The world has changed a lot in the 23 centuries since then. But what hasn't changed is that sometimes you don't have any good choices. You're left deciding which bad choice is the best.

Having stomach surgery is an extreme treatment. But being greatly overweight counts as an extreme illness. Sometimes surgery is the best choice of treatment. This chapter will tell you about the kinds of stomach surgery and their risks and successes.

KINDS OF SURGERY

People who are thinking about having surgery to help them lose weight have several stomach surgeries to choose from. The two most used in the United States are vertical banded gastroplasty and gastric bypass surgery. Both have the same goal: to make the stomach much smaller so that it holds very little food. Very little food means just that—right after surgery, the stomach holds less than 2 ounces. (After a few months, though, the stomach may be able to hold a little more food, sometimes as much as a small meal.) The idea is that a person who has the surgery will eat less and so lose weight.

Restriction Surgery

In a restriction surgery, the stomach is divided into two sections. The small pouch on top holds very little food, which must squeeze through a narrow passage to get to the rest of the stomach and then to the intestines.

One common restriction surgery is vertical banded gastroplasty. In this operation, the small upper pouch is created by stapling the stomach, leav-

---

TALKING ABOUT EATING AFTER STOMACH SURGERY

What kind of diet will I have to eat right after surgery?

For a few weeks after the surgery, you are on a liquid diet. Afterward, you slowly add foods such as soup and gelatin. Later, you add puréed food. After 6 weeks or so, you will slowly start eating regular food.

When can I return to my normal eating habits?

After surgery, you will never eat normally again. The amount of food you can eat at once will be small, and you'll need to eat very slowly. It's vital to chew, chew, chew, and then chew some more. You may not be able to tolerate certain foods.

What foods are most likely to cause me problems?

Most people are unable to eat red meats without vomiting. Some people can't eat chicken or turkey either. Bread and scrambled eggs can sometimes cause vomiting. Also, if you've had a gastric bypass, eating sweets and refined foods can cause dumping (weakness, sweating, upset stomach, diarrhea, and fainting).

ing only a small opening to the lower stomach. Often, the opening is reinforced with a band of a material that doesn't stretch. This narrow passage keeps the food from leaving the stomach too quickly.

In the name vertical banded gastroplasty, "vertical" refers to the direction of stapling, and "banded" refers to the nonstretching band that reinforces the narrow opening. "Gastroplasty" means reshaping the stomach, just as rhinoplasty means reshaping the nose.

Gastric Bypass Surgery

In gastric bypass surgery, most of the stomach is bypassed altogether. Instead, the food is rerouted to the small intestine.

The most common form of gastric bypass surgery goes by the exotic name Roux-en-Y bypass. In this operation the stomach is stapled to create a small pouch. A piece of small intestine joins this pouch to a later portion of the small intestine. Because the food bypasses the first part of the small intestine, it is not absorbed well. So people who have this operation tend to lose more weight.

Other Surgeries

In 1991, a National Institutes of Health Consensus Conference endorsed vertical banded gastroplasty and Roux-en-Y bypass as effective treatments for obesity.

But several other kinds of restriction surgeries and gastric bypasses are also done. For example, some surgeons use a ring instead of a band (vertical ring gastroplasty), and some staple horizontally instead of vertically (horizontal gastroplasty). Some surgeons cut and sew the stomach rather than stapling it to create a more secure pouch.

One promising new kind of restriction operation is called adjustable gastric banding. Instead of stapling the stomach, the surgeon cinches a silicone "belt" (called a band) around it. Later, if the passage to the lower stomach turns out to be too tight or too loose, the surgeon can easily inflate or deflate the band so that it's a perfect fit without further surgery. This surgery is often done "laparoscopically." That is, the surgeon makes only a small cut in the abdomen and does the surgery through a small tube. Because the incision is small, there should be less pain, less scarring, and quicker healing.

If you are thinking about having stomach surgery, ask the surgeon about the history of the procedure he or she suggests. When was it invented? How many people have had the surgery? Are there any published studies of how well it works? What experience has the surgeon had with the procedure?

GOOD EFFECTS OF STOMACH SURGERY

Most people who have stomach surgery lose weight, lots of it. Some people get down to a normal weight.

This large amount of weight loss has good effects on many aspects of health and social life. (These effects are not unique to stomach surgery. People who lose a lot of weight by any method would see good effects.)

- Glucose levels tend to drop in people with diabetes. Some people's glucose levels return to normal and stay there for many years.

- Blood pressure usually drops in people with high blood pressure. Some people's blood pressure returns to normal.

- Cholesterol levels may improve.

- Most people breathe and sleep better. For example, both asthma and sleep apnea may improve.

- People also can move more easily and with less pain. For people with arthritis, losing weight lightens the load on tender joints and so can greatly reduce pain and disability.

- Many people who were not able to work because of their weight can get jobs again after their surgery.

These good effects do more than just make a person feel better now. Bringing glucose levels down to normal or close to it should reduce complications later. Bringing blood pressure and cholesterol levels down reduces the risk of heart disease and stroke later. So surgery may help some people live longer and healthier lives.

Studies confirm that stomach surgery can take off a lot of weight. (See the boxes "Spotlight on Research: One Surgeon's Experience" and "Spotlight on Research: A Long-Term Study of Gastric Bypasses.") Even though weight starts creeping up again after a couple of years, the average person keeps a lot of weight off. People with diabetes seem to reap great benefits from stomach surgery. If these two studies are any guide, 50% to 90% of people no longer need to take any diabetes drugs. On the downside, most people didn't get to their ideal body weight. And sadly, the operation proved fatal for a few people.

THE DOWNSIDE OF STOMACH SURGERY

As with any surgery, some problems can occur right away. Stomach surgeries also affect the rest of your life. They change how you eat. Many people also get side effects.

Problems That Can Occur Right After Surgery

Stomach surgery carries a small risk of death (as does any surgery). The most common causes are infection caused by leaks from the stomach or intestines and blood clots in an artery in the lung.

Perhaps 1 in about 20 people gets an infected wound.

Side Effects That Show Up Later

Serious side effects are rare after stomach surgery, but do sometimes occur. Not every operation causes every side effect. Your surgeon can explain which side effects may occur with the surgery you are thinking of having. Side effects include:

- Vomiting (the most frequent side effect), usually caused by not chewing food long enough

- Stretching of the stomach, which allows more food in the stomach and so can lead to weight regain

- Staple leaks, which allow more food in the stomach and so can lead to weight regain

SPOTLIGHT ON RESEARCH
One Surgeon's Experience

Asurgeon performed 153 gastric bypass surgeries between 1975 and 1986 and reported the results in the *Journal of the American College of Nutrition* in 1994. All the patients either were at least 100 pounds above their ideal body weight or were at least double their ideal body weight. None had been able to keep weight off by other methods. Later patients got Roux-en-Y bypasses, while earlier patients got a different type of bypass.

After 5 years, 86 patients were still coming for their follow-up exams. Three people had died by then (one soon after surgery from a lung disease and two from cancer). The rest had stopped coming to appointments, and their fates were unknown.

The surgeon found that among his patients:

- Fifteen people had a complication from the surgery within a month.

- Six people got infections.

- At least 30 people had to go through a second operation to fix a problem caused by the first surgery.

- Average weight loss after 1 year was about 107 pounds.

- Average weight loss after 2 years was about 125 pounds.

- After 2 years, weight started creeping back up, and the average weight regain was 43 pounds. So the net weight lost and kept off was 82 pounds.

- Of the 86 people followed long term, 10 had been on diabetes drugs before surgery. Only 5 were on any diabetes drugs 5 years later. Presumably, weight loss improved glucose levels in the other 5 so much that they no longer needed diabetes drugs. Similarly, heart disease and high blood pressure improved in the people who had had them before surgery.

This study shows that even though some weight comes back, the average person keeps off a lot of pounds and enjoys better health.

SPOTLIGHT ON RESEARCH
A Long-Term Study of Gastric Bypasses

In a study published in 1995 in the *Annals of Surgery*, surgeons followed 608 very overweight people who had gastric bypasses. A few were followed for as long as 14 years. Before surgery, 165 of these people had type 2 diabetes, and another 165 had impaired glucose tolerance. (That is, their glucose levels were higher than normal, but below the cutoff for diabetes.) The researchers found that:

- Average weight loss after 1 year was 112 pounds.

- People hit their lowest weight about 2 years after surgery.

- Nine people (1.5%) died soon after the operation.

- Average body mass index started at 49.7, dropped to 31.5 by 5 years after surgery, and then rose to 34.7 by 10 years after surgery.

- Glucose levels began falling within days of surgery, even before much weight had been lost.

- Of the people with diabetes or impaired glucose tolerance, glucose levels dropped to normal in 91% of them and stayed there.

- Three-quarters of the people with high blood pressure had normal blood pressure after surgery.

- Many other health problems—including sleep apnea, snoring, asthma, limitations in movement due to arthritis, and infertility—improved in most people.

This study shows that stomach surgery improves weight-related health problems in most people and that people lose a lot of weight.

- "Dumping," that is, weakness, sweating, upset stomach, diarrhea, and fainting

- Lactose intolerance, that is, you lose the ability to digest milk products

- Vitamin deficiencies or even malnutrition from not getting enough nourishment

- Mineral deficiencies, including calcium and iron deficiencies, which can lead to fragile bones and anemia

- Ulcers

- Erosion (break down) of the band after vertical banded gastroplasty

- Sudden blockage of the passage to the lower stomach

Some side effects are the result of losing large amounts of weight. They would be likely to occur if a person lost that much weight by any method. These include:

- Loose skin

- Gallstones (see Chapter 4)

- Disappointment if the person thought losing weight would improve his or her marriage or win more friends

In addition, sometimes the surgery fails, and the person may need more surgery. And some people defeat the purpose of the operation by eating lots of soft or liquid high-calorie foods such as cheese, candy, ice cream, alcohol, and sugared soft drinks.

Obesity-Related Problems

Sometimes, an obesity-related problem may not go away after a person loses a lot of weight. For example, even though most people see a big improvement in their blood pressure after surgery, some people still have high blood pressure. So although it's a good bet your health will be better after surgery, there's no guarantee.

A NEW LIFE AFTER SURGERY

Hazel Gilberti weighed 270 pounds when she went to a surgeon to talk about having a gastric bypass done. But that wasn't her top weight; she had dieted down from 287—"just out of embarrassment"—in preparation for the visit.

Gilberti had been considering a gastric bypass for years. She finally decided to explore the option. "I was approaching my 50th birthday. This was my birthday present to myself."

Gilberti went to support groups to learn about the surgery and what to expect. "I knew how sick I might be, how intolerant of foods I might be." She felt prepared for the worst and decided to go ahead. She had more than a few days of wishing she hadn't.

"They were not whistlin' Dixie. It was absolutely brutal," she says. "I've had two major surgeries since that were nothing as painful as the bypass." She was in the hospital for 9 days and says it took her 2 months before she felt human again.

The weight didn't melt off, but after 3 months Gilberti noticed she had dropped a few sizes. In the first year, she lost over 100 pounds—and did a lot of shopping. "I got my ears pierced, I bought $300 worth of make-up, I had my hair styled. I used to wear polyester pants and polyester smock tops because they fit. I'd never been able to buy a designer outfit. My first full outfit was a designer outfit. It was the thrill of my life, because it was not a plus size."

Her surgery was in the late 1980s. Today, she weighs 150. She hasn't taken insulin since the day of her surgery. She doesn't check her blood glucose anymore; yearly tests done by her doctor show that her blood glucose levels are normal.

Although she can eat bigger meals now (the pouch stretches some with time), there are still foods she can't tolerate. "I don't do lots of meat or dairy products. Animal fats and refined sugars act as irritants. I have a better tolerance of pastas and salads." Even though the surgery forces her to eat healthy foods, keeping weight down is

A NEW LIFE AFTER SURGERY *Continued*

still a struggle. "The surgery is great for a year," Gilberti says. "It gets 100 pounds off—it's almost a guarantee, if you adhere to the program. But it's only a working tool.

"Your appetite does increase as you get further away from the surgery. After about a year, you can suddenly tolerate a banana, popcorn, small meals. That's when you have to be watchful. The surgery corrects the size of your stomach, but it doesn't stop the brain from all the craving."

Despite the difficult days after the surgery and the continuing struggle to maintain her weight, Gilberti says the surgery was worth it. "I would do it again. It's awful to say, but I feel like a normal person because I'm normal size. I can go to regular-size stores and buy clothes, I fit in bus seats and airplane seats, I'm not embarrassed by my size anymore."

THE GOOD CANDIDATE

A good candidate for stomach surgery is a person for whom the risks of death and side effects from surgery are less than the risks of staying greatly overweight.

According to the 1996 guidelines of the American Obesity Association and Shape Up America!, stomach surgery is an option when a person is at extremely high health risk from overweight. For a person with diabetes, that means a body mass index (see Chapter 1) higher than 35.

These guidelines also say that no weight-loss program, including stomach surgery, should be undertaken by pregnant women, people with unstable medical or mental conditions, people who have fatal diseases, or people with eating disorders.

Some surgeons may do the surgery only on people who have tried many other weight-loss methods and failed.

The Skinny on Chapter

16

▶ Stomach surgery is a life-changing operation in both good and bad ways.

▶ Stomach surgeries reduce the size of the stomach so that it holds less food.

▶ The two most common stomach surgeries are vertical banded gastroplasty and gastric bypass surgery.

▶ Death from stomach surgery is rare.

▶ Side effects are common after stomach surgery and include vomiting, gallstones, and vitamin deficiencies.

▶ People who have weight-related health problems usually see them improve or even go away after stomach surgery.

▶ In particular, diabetes often improves, and some people are able to get off diabetes drugs.

▶ The risks of stomach surgery must be weighed against the risks of staying overweight. For people with diabetes, the risks of obesity may outweigh the risks of surgery if their body mass index is above 35.

Your Weight-Loss Program Must Coordinate With Your Diabetes Care.

6

The sixth key to weight loss is that you can't treat your weight-loss program as something separate and apart from your diabetes care. Diabetes affects your weight loss. Weight loss in turn affects your diabetes. Losing weight will bring your glucose level down, and it may change the dose of diabetes drugs you need. Your diabetes treatment can speed or slow your weight loss.

Knowing what kind of diabetes you have and what that means for your weight-loss program prepares you for the twists and turns your weight-loss program may take. Knowledge is power.

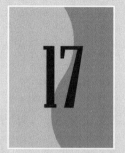

17

Different forms of diabetes have different effects on weight.

What You Need to Know About Diabetes and Weight

"How many legs does a dog have if you call a tail a leg?" Abraham Lincoln supposedly enjoyed asking. The answer to the riddle is four. Why? Because calling a tail a leg doesn't make it one.

How many kinds of diabetes are there? No one quite knows. Forms of diabetes are not as easy to tell apart as legs and tails. Currently, diabetes is separated into four groups:

- Diabetes caused by too little secretion of insulin (type 1 diabetes)

- Diabetes caused by resistance to the effects of insulin (type 2 diabetes)

- Diabetes that starts during pregnancy (gestational diabetes)

- Other types (a grab bag of disorders of too-high glucose levels with known causes)

But it's certainly possible that some tails—and maybe even some ears—are being mislabeled as legs. As doctors learn more about diabetes, some people's diagnoses will change. It will be years before doctors sort out all the kinds of diabetes and can label each person with accuracy.

Although there may be dozens of kinds of diabetes, you probably have type 1 or type 2. Most people with diabetes in the United States do. That's the main reason that the forms in the "other types" group are so little known.

This chapter will tell you about the differences among the various types of diabetes, especially type 1 and type 2. You'll learn how the type of diabetes you have is likely to affect your weight.

DIAGNOSIS OF DIABETES

The American Diabetes Association defines three ways to diagnose type 1 and type 2 diabetes in adults. These are based on three tests for glucose:

- In a blood glucose test, your glucose level is measured at some random time, perhaps as part of a general blood test.

- In a fasting blood glucose test, you fast for at least 8 hours before your glucose is tested.

- In an oral glucose tolerance test, you fast for 10 hours overnight. Your fasting blood glucose is measured, and then you drink 75 grams of a glucose solution. The glucose level in your blood is then measured every 30 or 60 minutes for as many as five times.

You have diabetes if you meet just one of the following and then have the result confirmed by a second test on a different day:

- Your random blood glucose level is higher than 200 mg/dl and you have symptoms such as being very hungry or thirsty, having to urinate often, and losing weight.

- Your fasting blood glucose level is higher than 126 mg/dl.

- Your glucose level is higher than 200 mg/dl at the 2-hour point during an oral glucose tolerance test.

DIABETES COMPLICATIONS

In all forms of diabetes, glucose levels are too high. In the normal body, cells take glucose from the blood to use as fuel. In diabetes, cells take up glucose less readily. The reasons why vary from type to type. But the results are the same:

- Your body loses glucose by adding it to urine. With time, kidney disease may develop.

- Glucose coats cells and proteins in the blood. These cells then don't work well. Depending on where they are, they can clog your blood vessels or damage your nerve cells.

- High glucose levels provide a banquet for bacteria and fungi, which can increase the number of infections.

As a result, people whose glucose levels remain high for a long time may get diabetic neuropathy (nerve disease), nephropathy (kidney disease), retinopathy (eye disease), heart and blood vessel disease, and frequent infections.

But scientists now know that most complications can be avoided by keeping glucose levels close to normal. The Diabetes Control and Complications Trial (DCCT) was a 10-year-long study of 1,441 people with type 1 diabetes. Some followed the standard treatment for diabetes. Others followed a stricter treatment. This included exercising, eating a better diet, testing their glucose often, and taking at least three insulin shots a day or using an insulin pump. The people on the stricter treatment, called tight control, kept their glucose levels closer to normal. In people who did not have complications at the start of the DCCT, those on tight control were far less likely to get eye, nerve, or kidney disease. In people who did have one or more of these complications already, the complications were far less likely to worsen in people on tight control.

Scientists believe the results apply to people with other kinds of diabetes as well. Most or all complications of diabetes are caused by too-high glucose levels. Keeping glucose tightly controlled can slow the development of complications and sometimes prevent them altogether.

TYPE 1 DIABETES

When insulin-producing cells in the pancreas are destroyed, usually by an immune reaction, type 1 diabetes is the result. About 980,000 people in the United States have type 1 diabetes. Of these, about 123,000 are younger than 18. Type 1 diabetes often strikes at young ages, most commonly in childhood or adolescence, but it can occur later.

Immune-Mediated Diabetes

By far, the most common form of type 1 diabetes is immune-mediated diabetes. It is caused by an overzealous immune system. The immune system is supposed to find and destroy bacteria, viruses, fungi, and other invaders that breach the defenses of the body. But in immune-mediated diabetes, the body mounts an autoimmune attack (an attack on its own tissues) against the beta cells in the pancreas, the cells that produce insulin. When no beta cells are left, the person must inject insulin to replace what is no longer being made.

Former names for immune-mediated diabetes include insulin-dependent diabetes and juvenile diabetes.

Idiopathic Type 1 Diabetes

In idiopathic type 1 diabetes, insulin-producing cells are destroyed, but doctors don't know why. Idiopathic type 1 diabetes is uncommon and runs in families.

Polyglandular Autoimmune Syndromes

Some people's immune systems are more easily aroused than other people's. As a result, autoimmune diseases often occur in clusters. People with immune-mediated diabetes are especially prone to autoimmune diseases of organs of the endocrine system. In addition to diabetes, they may also have Addison's disease (autoimmune disease of the adrenal glands), thyroid disease, anemia, loss of skin color, or loss of hair. The peak age for getting immune-mediated diabetes as part of a cluster of immune diseases is 30 to 40.

Weight and Type 1 Diabetes

The stereotype of a person with type 1 diabetes is someone who is thin or even scrawny. Like many stereotypes, this one is often not true. People whose glucose is badly controlled are sometimes thin because their cells are absorbing little glucose. Glucose goes into the urine instead. Calories get flushed away instead of being used by the body.

But doctors are learning more about keeping diabetes under good control. As a result, they are finding that people with type 1 diabetes are now often normal weight or even overweight.

WHAT A DIFFERENCE A DAY MAKES

"We went to the zoo, and I was walking around. I got dizzy and kind of nauseous," says Stephan Windrum. "The next day I went to the doctor to find out about it, and he found sugar in my urine."

Learning he had diabetes was a wake-up call for Windrum. "It changed my whole way of living," he says. "I quit smoking the day I found out." Despite weighing 308 pounds, he had never tried to lose weight before. But he wanted to live. He began limiting his food intake to 1,800 calories a day. To deal with his hunger, he keeps sugarless gum at work and sometimes takes an apple or orange to munch on. He is also learning more about food and nutrition and becoming savvy at reading labels. For example, he bought some "sugar-free" candies, thinking that he wouldn't have to limit how many he ate. When they gave him a lot of gas, he asked his dietitian about them. He found out that candies with so-called sugar alcohols in them have lots of calories and can cause intestinal side effects. (For more about sugar alcohols, see Chapter 8.)

His new eating habits have done the trick for him. His original weight goal was 250. But he has now lost 65 pounds and is shooting for 200. Now, he says, "I have a lot more energy. I can run and breathe, and I don't gasp for air anymore."

You read earlier in this chapter about the DCCT. This study showed that tight control could slow or prevent many complications in people with type 1 diabetes. But people gained an average of 10 pounds. The DCCT scientists studied this side effect in more detail and published the results in *Diabetes Care* in 1995. They found that at the start of the DCCT, between 5% and 9% of the subjects were overweight. But by the time the study ended, one in three people on tight control was overweight vs. only one in five of those on standard therapy.

The researchers compared these rates with the rate of overweight in Americans in general. The 19% obesity rate of people on standard treatment was close to the 23% rate of Americans of the same age and sex. But the 33% rate among the people on tight control was much higher.

When researchers looked at the entire course of the study, rates of overweight were even higher. A total of 42% of people on tight control had been overweight at some time during the study, but only 27% of people on standard therapy had. These results show clearly that with modern methods of controlling diabetes, people with type 1 diabetes can become overweight.

This study and others link overweight in people with type 1 diabetes with tight control. For example, a 1990 study in *Diabetes Care* found that for each 1% decrease in glycated hemoglobin, weight increased by almost 2 pounds.

TYPE 2 DIABETES

Type 2 is in some ways much more complex than type 1 diabetes. It appears to have many, many causes, sometimes more than one in a single person.

At the root, though, all people with type 2 diabetes share some features in common. Their bodies are still able to make insulin (although not as much as they need). But their cells are not able to use it as well as they should. So their cells do not take in enough glucose from the blood.

Insulin's job is to help cells extract glucose from blood. Cells have proteins on their surface that fit together with insulin like puzzle pieces. When an insulin molecule snaps into one of these proteins, called receptors, the cell membrane opens to admit glucose. In most people with type 2 diabetes, something goes wrong with this process. Usually, the cell resists taking in glucose even though the insulin and its receptor have linked. Other people have abnormal receptors that don't work right. And a few people have abnormal insulin molecules that don't fit into the receptor correctly.

All these problems are lumped together as "insulin resistance." But insulin resistance is not the sole problem in type 2 diabetes. Beta cells also do not work as well as they should and put out less insulin than is needed.

The first choice of therapy for type 2 diabetes is a combination of exercise, a healthful diet, and weight loss. Sometimes, these are not enough by themselves. Then doctors usually add a diabetes pill. When diabetes pills, too, are not enough, doctors may switch the person to insulin, combine insulin shots and a diabetes pill, or combine different types of diabetes pills.

In the United States, type 2 diabetes is usually a disease of middle age and older. Perhaps 15 million Americans have type 2 diabetes. Some previous names you may have heard for type 2 diabetes are non-insulin-dependent diabetes and adult-onset diabetes.

Weight and Type 2 Diabetes

Weight and type 2 diabetes intertwine tightly. People who are overweight are at much higher risk of getting type 2 diabetes, and most people who get type 2 diabetes, perhaps as many as 90%, are overweight. In addition, extra fat, particularly in the upper body, makes insulin resistance worse.

Losing weight has only good effects on type 2 diabetes. Weight loss boosts insulin sensitivity. Insulin binds better to its receptors on the cells, and the cells let in more glucose. As cells lose their resistance to insulin, the pancreas doesn't need to work as hard making the hormone.

All these good effects mean that weight loss improves glucose control. So after weight loss, a person with type 2 diabetes may be able to switch from insulin to diabetes pills or from diabetes pills to no drug at all. Complications are also less likely. Weight-related health problems, such as high blood pressure and joint pains, usually get better, too. For all these reasons, losing weight is one of the best treatments for type 2 diabetes.

Preventing Type 2 Diabetes

Scientists now know enough about type 2 diabetes to suppress and perhaps to prevent most cases. Research has shown that preventing obesity greatly delays and may even prevent the development of type 2 diabetes in monkeys. And there's no reason to believe that this is not true in humans as well. In fact, one of the aims of a large study called the Diabetes Prevention Program is to prove just that.

Measures to prevent type 2 diabetes are cheap enough for almost anyone to adopt, are safe enough for many people with health problems, and have mostly good side effects. These measures are the same lifestyle changes you need to make to keep your weight under control. And these changes can also help protect your family from getting diabetes later.

This is a great reason not to keep your weight loss efforts to yourself. Include your family in your exercise program, and make healthful meals for the whole family. You'll be giving them the best gift possible—a longer, healthier life.

PEOPLE AT RISK OF GETTING TYPE 2 DIABETES

Although healthful habits are a good idea for everyone, people who would benefit the most are those who are at the highest risk of getting type 2 diabetes:

- Brothers and sisters of people with type 2 diabetes
- Children of people with diabetes
- Parents of people with diabetes
- Women who've had gestational diabetes (diabetes that started during pregnancy)
- People who are overweight
- People who are sedentary
- American Indians, African-Americans, and Mexican-Americans

GESTATIONAL DIABETES

When someone who does not have diabetes gets diabetes while pregnant, she is said to have gestational diabetes. Almost always, it goes away after the baby is born. But every so often, it doesn't, and the person is then diagnosed with one of the other forms of diabetes.

Gestational diabetes is caused by a combination of insulin resistance and too-low insulin production. A pregnant woman's body makes hormones that help the fetus develop. But these hormones also have an effect on the woman. They prevent her insulin from doing its job. When a woman cannot make enough extra insulin, her glucose levels rise, and she has gestational diabetes.

About 135,000 women in the United States get gestational diabetes each year. Scientists guess that 2% to 12% of pregnant women are affected. This range spans such a large interval because the risk of getting gestational diabetes varies from place to place and among ethnic groups. Risk factors for gestational diabetes include being older, having relatives with diabetes, or being overweight.

The first therapy tried is usually a combination of exercise and a special diet. The goals of therapy are to reduce glucose levels while allowing the woman to gain weight and the fetus to grow correctly. If exercise and the special diet fail at these goals, then insulin shots are the next step.

Weight and Gestational Diabetes

Being overweight makes a woman more likely to get gestational diabetes, but plenty of normal-weight women get it, too. No matter what a woman weighs, she still needs to gain some weight during pregnancy. But the amount that's best to gain is lower in heavier women. As discussed in Chapter 2, your doctor can tell you how much weight you should gain during pregnancy.

A healthy fetus depends on more than the mother gaining the right amount of weight. Just as vital is that the woman keep her glucose in good control. Your doctor's suggestions will be based on finding a balance between good glucose control and good weight gain (not too little, not too much).

Women who've had gestational diabetes have a high chance of getting type 2 diabetes later. But they can cut their risk in half by:

- Staying at a normal weight (or losing weight if they are overweight)
- Eating a diet based on the Food Guide Pyramid
- Exercising regularly

OTHER FORMS OF DIABETES

The last category of diabetes is like the junk drawer in your kitchen. It contains all the odds and ends that didn't fit anywhere else. Here are just a few examples:

- Some people have genetic mutations that reduce the amount of insulin their beta cells can make.
- Some people get diabetes because their pancreas has been damaged or destroyed. For example, it may have been damaged in an accident or by cancer or cystic fibrosis.
- In rare cases, drugs can cause diabetes.
- Diabetes occurs more often than usual in people with certain genetic diseases and syndromes, including Down's syndrome and Huntington's disease (the disease that killed Woody Guthrie).

Obesity often accompanies some of these forms of diabetes.

DO YOU NEED TO KNOW WHICH TYPE YOU HAVE?

Sometimes, it's clear which form of diabetes a person has. Sometimes, it's pretty murky.

Not having a precise diagnosis can be stressful; having one of the unnamed "other" forms of diabetes can be awkward. In either case, you may find it hard to talk about your diabetes with other people when you can't put a name to it. You may have trouble learning more about your condition because almost all diabetes information (including this book) is aimed at people who are known to have type 1 or type 2 diabetes. You may also have problems when you apply for insurance or change doctors.

But these problems should not get in the way of your doctor's care. No matter what kind of diabetes you have, your treatment plan should be designed just for you. It should be aimed at lowering your glucose levels so that you feel better and get fewer complications later.

The Skinny on Chapter

17

▶ Diabetes is divided into four major groups: type 1, type 2, gestational, and other kinds.

▶ Almost everyone with diabetes in the United States has type 1 or type 2.

▶ Diabetes is diagnosed when a blood glucose test shows that glucose is unusually high.

▶ High glucose levels can damage the nerves, kidneys, eyes, heart, and blood vessels.

▶ Immune-mediated type 1 diabetes results when the immune system destroys the insulin-making beta cells of the pancreas.

▶ People with immune-mediated diabetes are at higher risk of getting other autoimmune diseases as well.

▶ Idiopathic type 1 diabetes results when the beta cells are destroyed for an unknown reason.

▶ Once, poor control meant most people with type 1 diabetes were lean. But today, they can sometimes be overweight.

▶ Type 2 diabetes results when cells aren't able to use glucose as well as they should and can't put out enough insulin to make up for this problem.

▶ Insulin resistance means that cells don't take in enough glucose even though there's insulin in the blood.

▶ Weight and diabetes are intertwined. Greater weight leads to greater insulin resistance, while weight loss improves diabetes control.

▶ Gestational diabetes results when insulin resistance raises the need for insulin during pregnancy and the pancreas cannot keep up with the extra demand.

▶ Many other forms of diabetes exist.

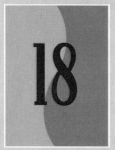

18

Diabetes and your
diabetes treatments
affect how easily you
lose weight.

How Diabetes Hinders and Helps Your Weight-Loss Program

Do you have one of THOSE closets? The kind where wrapping paper rolls tumble in every direction when you open the door, and reaching the guest linens requires half an hour of unpacking? Trying to lose weight when you have diabetes can be like dealing with one of those closets. The relations between diabetes and weight loss are so twisted and tangled that any change in one can involve the other.

This chapter will show you some of the ways that your weight, your weight-loss efforts, your diabetes, and your diabetes treatments interact. Little research has been done on some of these interactions, so you'll see there are still plenty of holes in our knowledge.

EFFECTS OF DIABETES AND DIABETES TREATMENTS ON WEIGHT

Some treatments that help lower glucose levels also affect weight and appetite.

Exercise and a Reduced-Calorie Diet

The first choice of therapy for type 2 diabetes is exercise and good eating habits. These are usually prescribed for people with type 1 diabetes as well. And they are also the best treatments for overweight. So in this case, there's no conflict at all between your diabetes treatment plan and your weight-loss program.

A study in *Diabetes Care* in 1994 looked at the effects of a reduced-calorie diet and exercise on glucose control. The researchers reviewed the medical charts of 408 men and 244 women with type 2 diabetes who had attended a 26-day health program. (The program aimed to improve people's health by helping them become active, restrict fat intake, and reduce stress.) The subjects ranged in age from 19 to 83. Each day, they walked or did other aerobic exercise. All ate a diet that was high in fiber and complex carbohydrates and that had fewer than 10% of its calories from fat. Because of the bulkiness of this diet, people tended to eat fewer calories than before.

At the end of the program, everyone had greatly improved heart disease risk factors and diabetes control:

- Fasting glucose levels fell.

- Cholesterol and triglyceride levels and blood pressure also fell.

- At the beginning of the program, 409 people were taking insulin or diabetes pills. But at the end, only 191 were.

- Of the 319 people who'd been on high blood pressure pills, a third were able to stop.

- Even though the people spent only 26 days at the health center, weight dropped an average of about 10 pounds.

Most people continued to exercise and follow the low-fat, high-complex-carbohydrate diet for at least 2 years afterward, and their diabetes stayed in control.

Clearly, exercise plus a healthful, low-fat diet works both to improve diabetes and to help people lose weight. But this study also found that people who were taking insulin at the start got less benefit than the others. The researchers interpreted this difference to mean that people who change their habits early in the course of their diabetes (when they have not yet started insulin) reap bigger gains than people who wait until their diabetes gets out of hand. Still, everyone got some good from adopting more-healthful habits.

HOW DIABETES AFFECTS MEAL PLANNING

I know that a diet based on the Food Guide Pyramid is best for both people with diabetes and those without. Does that mean I can ignore my diabetes when planning meals?

No. Because you have diabetes, you need to keep two other factors in mind. In general, people with diabetes keep their glucose under best control if:

- They eat the same number of calories at the same time each day.

- They plan the timing (and possibly the content) of their meals to prevent sudden upswings in glucose levels.

So is it okay to eat just dinner or just lunch and dinner as long as I eat the same number of calories each day?

Eating just one or two large meals a day is probably the worst choice you can make. Getting an entire day's worth of calories at once sends your glucose level soaring. In contrast, eating many smaller meals means that a smaller dose of carbohydrates enters your system each time. So your glucose stays on a more even keel.

It is thought that spreading out the absorption of carbohydrates may have several good effects:

- Your body may need less insulin to handle your meals.

- Your average glucose level over time may be lower.

- Less cholesterol may be produced.

- You don't get as hungry, so it may be easier not to overeat.

To help you space out your carbohydrates, your diabetes meal plan may call for three meals and three snacks each day.

HOW DIABETES AFFECTS MEAL PLANNING *Continued*

What if I want to eat four or five meals a day instead of just three?

If your schedule lets you eat more than three meals a day, you may be better off. Check with your dietitian. He or she can help you choose when to eat and how to distribute your calorie allotment for each day. Remember, eating more meals each day doesn't mean eating more calories each day.

Do I need to have regular meals if I don't use insulin?

Yes. If you use diet and exercise alone to control your diabetes, you have fewer tools for controlling your glucose. Consistent mealtimes and consistent calorie intake are two of the best ways you have to smooth out glucose spikes.

What if you take diabetes pills or the same insulin dose each day? Then each day they provide the same glucose-lowering effect at the same times. You want the glucose from your meal to enter your bloodstream when the drugs are taking effect. If you don't time your meal correctly or if you eat more or less food than your diabetes drug can handle, your glucose level may fall too low or rise too high.

What if you use insulin and are on tight control? If you adjust your insulin dose based on how much you plan to exercise and to eat, you have more freedom. Then you don't have to match your meal to your drug dose and schedule. You can match your drug dose and schedule to your expected meal, if you prefer.

In this case, it's okay to eat somewhat more or less than usual or eat at a different time—as long as you plan ahead and adjust your dose of insulin to the size and time of the upcoming meal. But keep in mind that losing weight depends on sticking to a reduced-calorie food plan. If you routinely take extra insulin to allow yourself to eat more food while keeping your glucose controlled, you're likely to gain weight, not lose it.

Diabetes and Changes in Taste

Several research groups have found that people with diabetes lose some of their ability to smell and taste. Various researchers have suggested that changes are due to dry mouth (which is more frequent in people with diabetes and can affect the sense of taste), diabetic nerve disease, or a defect in the taste buds.

Changes in taste do not directly affect weight. But because taste is such an important quality of food, changes in taste can make nutritious foods seem less appealing. If taste changes possibly due to diabetes or diabetes treatments are bothering you, here are some things to try:

- See your dentist. Diabetes makes gum disease, infections, and dry mouth more likely, and one of these might be the cause of your taste problems.

- If you've recently started a new drug and think it is to blame, wait a bit. Some side effects improve after you've taken the drug for a while.

- If a drug continues to affect the way foods taste, ask your doctor about switching to a different drug.

- If dry mouth is your problem, sugar-free gum or sugar-free hard candy can make your mouth water.

- Chew food well. Doing so can increase the amount of flavor that you taste.

- Alternate between foods. The contrast will make each food seem more flavorful.

- Choose foods with a variety of textures.

- Let foods cool down or warm up a bit before eating. The flavor will become stronger.

Diabetes Pills

This section will cover only pills that can be prescribed in the United States, and only U.S. brand names will be listed.

Sulfonylureas. Until December 1994, the only diabetes pills approved for use in the United States were the sulfonylureas. This class of drugs includes tolbutamide (Oramide, Orinase), chlorpropamide (Diabinese), tolazamide (Tolamide, Tolinase), glipizide (Glucotrol), glyburide (also called glibenclamide; DiaBeta, Micronase), and glimepiride (Amaryl). They act by increasing insulin secretion. All these drugs may increase or decrease appetite and are thought to cause weight gain.

Metformin. Metformin (Glucophage) went on the market in the United States in 1995. (It has been used in other countries for about 40 years.) Its main action is to lower the amount of glucose your liver produces. Some people lose a bit of weight when they start taking metformin. Three percent of people who start metformin get a bad taste in their mouth, but it usually goes away.

Carbohydrase Inhibitors. Acarbose (Precose) went on the market in 1996. A similar drug called miglitol (Glyset) was approved by the FDA in 1996. Both slow the body's digestion of carbohydrates. Studies in rats found acarbose could reduce obesity, possibly by keeping some carbohydrates from being absorbed. These studies sparked hopes that acarbose could be used to treat human obesity. But these hopes were dashed in most human studies, which did not find this effect, even at large doses. But acarbose does not seem to increase weight, either.

Troglitazone. Troglitazone (Rezulin) went on the market in 1997. It's a drug that decreases insulin resistance. Most studies have found it to have no effect on weight. But it can improve some weight-related problems such as high fat in the blood (high triglycerides). So it may be a good choice of drug for people who are overweight and have heart disease risk factors.

If you are taking this drug, it is important that your doctor monitor you regularly for possible liver problems. This is done with a blood test for liver enzymes. The FDA has recommended monthly tests during the first 6 months of taking Rezulin, bimonthly tests for the next 6 months, and periodic tests thereafter.

Insulin

Like other hormones, insulin has many jobs. The job you usually hear about is getting cells to take in glucose. But insulin also has another important role: helping the body process fats. As part of this job, insulin appears to:

- Boost the production and storage of fat
- Boost the production of cholesterol
- Reduce the rate of fat burning
- Slow the breakdown of cholesterol

As you might guess, these actions of insulin are not useful to people who are overweight!

Insulin resistance often occurs in people with type 2 or gestational diabetes, and sometimes it develops in people with type 1 diabetes. When

SPOTLIGHT ON RESEARCH
Insulin Ups and Downs

A study published in *Diabetes Care* in 1993 showed clearly that people with type 2 diabetes are more likely to gain weight if they take insulin than if they take a diabetes pill. The researchers reviewed the medical charts of 27 American Indians who lived on the Navajo Reservation in Arizona. All had type 2 diabetes and had been taking insulin for at least 1 year. Over the years, their insulin dose had been increased and decreased as needed to control their diabetes.

The researchers found that when insulin doses were increasing, almost everyone gained weight. The average weight gain was about 7 pounds per year. On the other hand, when insulin doses were decreasing or when people stopped taking insulin, every single person lost weight. The average weight loss was about 11 pounds per year. The researchers then looked at weight changes in a similar group of 102 people who were not on insulin. These people did not gain weight. Also, 20 of the 27 subjects had been on diabetes pills before starting insulin. On average, they had lost weight during that time.

people's cells resist the effects of insulin, the body needs to make—or take in—extra insulin. This extra insulin in the bloodstream can encourage weight gain.

People with type 1 diabetes typically gain weight when they start a program of tight glucose control. Doctors believe this weight gain results from two factors. First, insulin encourages the body to put on fat. Second, tight control works to bring glucose levels close to normal. So the person's body processes food more normally. People in bad control can't absorb all the glucose from their food. They can lose hundreds of calories a day in their urine. But healthy people do absorb all the energy from food. As a result, they can gain weight.

DANGERS OF INSULIN UNDERDOSING AS A WEIGHT-LOSS METHOD

You've just seen that people in good control are able to use more calories from their food than people in bad control. Some people with diabetes use this fact to control their weight. They take too little insulin on purpose. The lower their insulin dose, the higher their glucose levels. They're absorbing fewer calories, allowing them to lose weight without watching what they eat.

This method is extremely dangerous. People in bad control may feel hungry and thirsty all the time, they may feel very tired, and their vision may blur. Not only is life less fun when you feel lousy and can't see well, but underdosing can also lead to complications, coma, and possibly even death.

Scientists do not know how many people with diabetes underdose their insulin. They believe the practice is more common in girls and young women with type 1 diabetes than in other people with diabetes. But estimates range widely. The study in *Diabetes Care* described in the box "Spotlight on Research: A Study of Underdosing" found that a third of women with type 1 diabetes let their control be bad on purpose to keep their weight down. Other studies have found rates ranging from 11% to 39%.

No matter what the true rate is, this practice does great harm. Diabetes goes out of control, and complications are more likely to develop.

If you sometimes skip insulin doses or take too little insulin, you should seek help, for two reasons:

SPOTLIGHT ON RESEARCH
A Study of Underdosing

A study in *Diabetes Care* in 1994 explored the problems caused by purposely taking too little insulin. In this study, Boston researchers surveyed 341 teenage girls and women who were between 13 and 60 years old and who had type 1 diabetes. All went to the same medical clinical for their diabetes care, and their average body mass index (BMI) was 24. The study's goal was to learn when, why, and how often women with diabetes skip taking their insulin, and what effects skipping had.

The researchers found that at some time, almost one-third of the women had taken less insulin than they were supposed to. Half of the women had done so to lose weight. Although the youngest women misused insulin the most often, underdosing occurred in all age groups. For example, among women under 30, 40% had underdosed; of women above the age of 46, 20% had. Underdosing was unrelated to the woman's BMI. Women of all weights, not just overweight women, underdosed sometimes.

Compared with the women who never took too little insulin, those who underdosed suffered medically:

- Their glucose control was worse.

- They were hospitalized more often for diabetes-related problems.

- They were more likely to have diabetic nerve disease.

- They were more likely to have diabetic eye disease.

These problems were extra likely in the women who misused insulin so that they could eat more without gaining weight.

- When you don't take good care of your diabetes, you're not just making yourself feel bad now. You're also setting yourself up for getting complications in the future.

- Some researchers have found that people who misuse insulin have a high rate of psychological problems. For example, they may have more trouble than usual dealing with having diabetes. Getting these problems treated will make you happier and help you stick to your diabetes care plan better.

DIABETES CREATES AN EXTRA LOAD

"Diabetes made me tired. I didn't want to exercise. I didn't want to do anything, really," says Isaiah Carpenter. He blames his insulin dose in part for weight he gained after his diagnosis. He explains what his doctor told him about insulin: "It increases your hunger, and it also chemically reduces the possibility of the body letting the fat go during metabolism. So the more insulin you take, the more weight you gain."

Diabetes had another effect on his weight as well. "With diabetes, my hands get cold fast. My feet are cold all the time, and the only time that they warm up is when I'm going to sleep," Carpenter says. Because he felt cold so often, and because he had to work outside in below-zero temperatures in the winter, he ate more food to help him stay warm.

When he weighed more than 400 pounds, he was taking 190 units of insulin a day. But when Carpenter joined a weight-loss clinic, they changed his medication so that he would no longer have to fight the effects of the insulin. He started on two diabetes pills, metformin and acarbose. These helped him control his diabetes better and let him cut way back on his insulin. The weight-loss clinic also started him walking every day and put him on weight-loss drugs. A year later, he had lost 65 pounds and was continuing to lose weight.

EFFECTS OF WEIGHT LOSS ON DIABETES

Just as diabetes and its treatments affect weight loss, your weight loss can affect your diabetes.

Effects on People Who Take Diabetes Pills

Although the sulfonylureas, metformin, acarbose, and troglitazone work in different ways, they do share one feature. They work best when people follow their diabetes diet. In addition, when people gain weight, their glucose levels often rise. Then pills that formerly kept glucose in good control may no longer be able to do so.

As you lose weight, your diabetes pills will work better. Your doctor may then put you on a lower dose or even say you can stop taking them altogether.

Effects on People Who Take Insulin

A larger body usually requires more insulin. Not only are there more cells that need insulin to help them take in glucose, but cells also seem less willing to accept glucose. So the heavier you are, the less likely it is that your body can make enough insulin to meet its own needs.

As with diabetes pills, if you lose weight, you will likely be able to lower your dose of insulin. To avoid problems, wait until your glucose improves to cut back on your insulin. Your glucose levels can go too high if you cut your insulin first because you expect your glucose to drop. If you have type 2 diabetes, your glucose level may improve so much that your doctor may switch you to diabetes pills.

Effects on Your Pocketbook

A study in *Preventive Medicine* in 1995 looked at how much people could save on diabetes drugs by losing weight. The subjects were 32 people between 40 and 70 years old. All had type 2 diabetes and body mass indexes (see Chapter 1) of 30 to 40. On average, their diabetes and high blood pressure drugs and supplies (such as syringes and test strips) cost $63.30 a month.

Then the people went on a very-low-calorie diet for 12 weeks. They lost an average of about 34 pounds. One year later, they had kept off an average of 20 pounds. Their glucose control and blood pressure improved. As a result, at the 1-year mark, they averaged only $32.40 per month on diabetes and blood pressure drugs and supplies. One man whose drugs had cost $184.90 every month no longer needed **any** blood pressure or diabetes drugs after losing weight. Of course, the added costs of the very-low-calorie diet might balance out the savings on drugs and supplies, unless the weight loss is maintained for a good while.

Weight loss can pay off!

The Skinny on Chapter

▶ Diabetes and diabetes treatments can affect your weight and weight-loss efforts. Your weight and weight-loss efforts can affect your diabetes and diabetes treatment.

▶ Exercising and eating a reduced-calorie diet are the best treatments for both type 2 diabetes and overweight.

▶ Losing weight can improve glucose levels and heart disease risk factors.

▶ Diabetes itself, as well as some diabetes pills, sometimes affects people's appetite or sense of taste. When nutritious foods lose their appeal, sticking to a weight-loss plan is harder.

▶ People who take sulfonylurea diabetes pills sometimes gain weight.

▶ People who take metformin sometimes lose weight.

▶ Troglitazone and acarbose appear not to affect weight.

▶ Insulin increases the production of fat and cholesterol and slows fat burning.

▶ Some people take too little insulin as a way to lose weight.

▶ Underdosing insulin is a very bad idea. It causes poor control, which causes unpleasant symptoms now and leads to earlier and more complications.

▶ When people lose weight, they are often able to reduce their dose of diabetes drug.

▶ After weight loss, people with type 2 diabetes may be able to switch from insulin to pills, or from insulin or pills to nothing at all.

Permanent Weight Loss Requires That You Change Your Lifestyle for Good.

7

The seventh and final key to losing weight is that a healthful diet and a more active lifestyle need to become ingrained habits. You can't put aside healthful behaviors when you've lost your excess weight the way you put away your winter coat when spring comes. Preventing weight regain is possible; many people do manage to do it. But you must fight your own body, which rebels at losing fat and which tries hard to get its fat back. You also have to fight your mind, which may use eating or sedentary pursuits such as watching TV to comfort itself or avoid confronting a problem. Many methods can help you stick to your new habits and prevent relapses.

CHAPTER

19

Good health habits—
such as brushing your
teeth, checking your
shoes for pebbles, and
eating right and
exercising—help you
most when you
practice them every
day.

The Need for Constant Vigilance

In life, sometimes you struggle mightily to surmount a towering problem—and once you achieve the peak, you discover you're only in the foothills of the real challenge. You grit your teeth and put up with high school's hair codes, restroom use restrictions, and useless assemblies—only to find at your first job that the rules are even sillier and the meetings even more snooze-inducing. You search long and hard for someone with the qualities you want in a wife or husband—and then learn that household harmony means coming to agreements about money, curtain colors, mealtimes, laundry frequency, and hundreds of other details. You get your toddler to sleep through the night—and then he discovers the word "no."

For many people, losing weight is like this. People expect losing weight to be a challenge. What comes as a surprise is that keeping it off is actually the hard part. Chapter 20 will discuss why and how people regain weight after losing it. But first, in this chapter, you'll find out how big the problem of weight regain is and learn many methods to make it easier to keep weight off for the long term.

WHAT HAPPENS DURING AND AFTER WEIGHT LOSS

Weight loss in study after study tends to follow the same depressing path. People lose weight for a while, perhaps 6 months or so. Then weight loss tapers off or stops. Most people then start regaining weight. After a year, about two-thirds of the weight has come back. After 5 years, almost all has.

This pattern may strike you as odd. If someone keeps eating a reduced-calorie diet, shouldn't weight keep dropping?

The reason it doesn't is that body weight is a balance between calories taken in and calories used up. A person at a steady weight is taking in enough calories to maintain the body, but not enough to put on weight. (Or, looked at in another way, the person is taking in few enough calories to prevent weight gain, but not few enough to lose weight.)

Think about a person at a stable weight who is eating 2,500 calories a day and then cuts back to 2,000 calories. At first, the person is eating too little food to maintain that weight. So weight comes off. But smaller bodies, like smaller cars, need less fuel than larger ones. After weight loss, the body may also work more efficiently. So as the person's body gets smaller, it needs fewer calories. Finally, the person reaches a weight that can be maintained on 2,000 calories. Weight loss stops. Calories are again in balance.

What happens next is the surprise. For most people, weight starts creeping up again. Rebound occurs for many reasons. Preventing it is the secret to lasting weight loss. Scientists believe that beating rebound depends on sticking with what helped you take the weight off in the first place. It has been said that the price of leanness is eternal vigilance. Continuing to restrict calorie intake is vital.

Also, if you are not already exercising, starting now is a good idea. Exercise helps to keep weight from coming back.

EXERCISE IN WEIGHT-LOSS MAINTENANCE

Exercise and a reduced-calorie diet have interlocking roles in weight loss. Cutting calories is the best way to take weight off. But for various reasons, weight tends to creep back up. Exercise, on the other hand, is not so good for helping people lose weight. It just doesn't burn enough

TIPS FOR STICKING WITH AN EXERCISE PROGRAM

Clearly, starting and staying with an exercise program can make a big difference in how much weight you keep off. But how do you keep exercising week after week and month after month?

Experts believe sticking with an exercise program is easier if you:

- Vary your activities so that you won't get bored or overstress yourself.

- Choose activities that are unlikely to injure you.

- Exercise with a group.

- Choose activities that are fun.

- Choose activities that mesh with your life—that you can do with small children in tow, for example, or in a climate with 6 months of winter.

- Set specific goals and have a plan for reaching them.

- Be alert to exercise's good effects on you—how many stairs you can climb, for example, or how long you can dig in your garden without taking a break.

- Ask your friends and family members for encouragement and support.

- Keep a record, such as a chart or notebook, of your exercise so that you can see how you're doing.

- Play music while you exercise.

Continued

STICKING WITH AN EXERCISE PROGRAM *Continued*

- Find a role model—someone who has similar constraints on his or her life but is able to stick with an exercise program.

- Schedule a time in your day for exercise just as you plan time to eat, sleep, and read the paper.

- Don't overdo it.

It's also important to keep in mind that people vary in how quickly they build muscle and improve fitness. It may take 2 to 3 months before you notice any changes. Sometimes, people exercise for a few weeks and then quit because they don't think it's working. In fact, they just didn't wait quite long enough.

---

calories. But exercise helps people keep from gaining (or regaining) weight. It also seems to slow or prevent weight gain as people get older. (See the box "Spotlight on Research: On the Beat.")

CHANGE YOUR THINKING

Two thousand years ago, Rabbi Hillel wrote, "If I am not for myself, who is for me? And if I am only for myself, what am I? If not now, when?" That in a nutshell summarizes the complex psychology of preventing weight regain. Weight loss has to be something you do for yourself, not for other people. Yet it can't be the center of your life. And you have to make keeping weight off part of every day. You can't put it off for another time.

Sounds like a tall order, doesn't it? But there are ways to make it easier.

Get in the Habit of Liking Yourself

Society places great importance on looks. So it's hard not to judge yourself by what you see in the mirror. But your worth as a person has nothing

SPOTLIGHT ON RESEARCH

On the Beat

An interesting study of the value of exercise in keeping weight off appeared in the *American Journal of Clinical Nutrition* in 1989. It focused on Boston policemen. All 184 men (no policewomen were included) were overweight and between 26 and 52 years old. All went to weekly sessions to learn about food choices and exercise. And all went on a reduced-calorie diet. Four diets were used, ranging from 420 to 1,000 calories a day. In addition, half the men were put in a supervised exercise program. These men had to exercise for 90 minutes three times a week. This amount of exercise burned an estimated extra 1,500 calories a week.

After the study was over (after 12 weeks in the pilot program and after 8 weeks in the main study), men in nonexercising groups had lost various amounts of weight, depending on which of the four diets they were on. But the men who exercised tended to lose more weight—about 32 pounds in the 12-week pilot program and roughly 27 pounds in the 8-week main study. The amount of weight lost did not depend on which diet the exercisers were assigned to.

The researchers followed the men for 3 years. By then, policemen who'd been in the nonexercising groups and continued not to exercise weighed almost as much as they had to start. But men in the exercise groups who continued to exercise kept all their weight off. Nonexercisers who had begun exercising kept off more weight, and exercisers who stopped gained back weight.

This study shows that exercising allowed men on moderate reduced-calorie diets to lose as much weight as men on very strict diets. Being policemen, the subjects may have had more self-discipline than average, and they probably benefited on the job from being lighter on their feet. So they may have had extra motivation to keep exercising. Whatever the reason, many of them did keep exercising, and these men were able to keep off all their lost weight.

to do with how tightly gravity binds you to the Earth. Losing weight will help you move around more freely and comfortably. It should improve your diabetes control and make your future healthier. But it won't make you kinder or wiser or braver.

Learning to like yourself is a very personal struggle. One starting step to liking yourself is to act as if you already do. For example:

- Don't beat yourself up over falling short of your goals. Some people let a minor boo-boo such as eating a piece of candy become an excuse for giving up altogether. Just as in horse-back riding, the best thing to do when you fall off a good-health program is to get right back on again.

- Set kind goals for yourself. "Even though I love chocolate cake, I'll never eat it again" is a cruel goal. "Because I love chocolate cake so much, I'll make a place in my meal plan for a slice at Sunday dinner" is a kind goal that allows you to treat yourself while staying within a healthful eating plan.

- Don't put life off until you're thinner. There's no reason to deny yourself a vacation or a pretty dress because you're overweight. When you've lost more weight, you can always get a new dress in a smaller size or take a more vigorous vacation.

- See yourself through the eyes of the people who love you. What do your friends and family see in you? Look hard to see those good qualities in yourself.

- Surround yourself with people who support you. For example, find a doctor who treats you with respect and is willing to help with your weight-control plan.

- Think positive thoughts about yourself. Some people's thoughts fall into ruts and hold them back. Each time something goes wrong, their mind starts replaying the same self-hating thoughts—"I'm so stupid!" or "I can't believe I did it again!" or "I never get anything right!" Listen to how you talk to yourself. Then get tough with bad thoughts. Each time one rears its ugly head, cut it off. Replace it with a more useful—and more truthful—thought. For example: "Everyone makes mistakes. This one's a doozy, so I can learn a lot from it!" or "I stuck to my meal plan last week. I can do it again."

Some researchers think that people who believe in themselves and their ability to change do better at weight loss than other people.

Find Ways to Motivate Yourself

In more brutal times, there were two ways to motivate a donkey to move: You could entice it with a carrot or beat it with a stick. Today, for animals and humans alike, the carrot approach is considered best.

Carrots. There are many ways to reward yourself for sticking to good habits:

- Choose activities and foods that you enjoy.

- Praise yourself each time you make a healthful food choice or work some extra activity into your life.

- When you meet a big goal (for example, 2 months without gaining back any weight), give yourself a present.

- Remind yourself often of the great progress you've made and how much better you feel. A pair of pants from before you

WHEN THE BABY CAME

Many people find the strength to do for their families what they can't do for themselves. Juanita Diaz, too, found it easier to stick to her diabetes treatment plan when she was pregnant. "During 1990, I lost 35 pounds, and I got pregnant," she says. "I did really well. The doctors thought that I wasn't going to have to take insulin, I was doing so well." She walked every day, and she watched everything she ate. She managed to avoid having to take insulin until she was in her eighth month of pregnancy.

Diaz lost her motivation as soon as her son was born. "After I delivered, that evening, I wanted chili dogs," she says. "My husband went after them for me." She has been on insulin since.

She still struggles with trying to watch her weight as well as she did when she was pregnant. "I could do it then because I had a purpose, my child," she says. "But I'm thinking, why can't I do it again?"

lost weight can be a visible reminder of how much weight you've lost.

Carrots and Sticks Together. Psychologists believe that mild punishment can work if combined with a reward. For example:

- Set aside a bit of money at the beginning of each week. If you meet your goals, then you get to have the money back. If not, then you must give it to a charity.

- Have a contest with someone else. For example, keep track of how many minutes each of you exercise. The loser each month has to pay the winner some money or do some chores for them.

- Make a chart or keep a diary. Each day, write in what you've done toward your goal. Squares with a lot of writing will make you feel good, and blank squares on the chart will make you feel bad, spurring you to have as few blank spots as possible.

Lose Weight for Yourself

Why and for whom are you trying to lose weight? Some people embark on a self-improvement program to please other people. Maybe they're tired of a husband's or wife's nagging. Or maybe their doctor told them to lose weight.

Other people start a weight-loss program because it's what they want to do. They want to improve their health or have more stamina for daily life.

Not surprisingly, people who set their own course in life instead of letting other people pressure them into things tend to be more creative in finding solutions for their problems and happier with the results.

Your reason for wanting to lose weight may affect your chances of success. Some psychologists believe that people are more likely to stick to behavioral changes when they themselves want the change. (See the box "Spotlight on Research: Losing for Yourself Not Others.")

Choose a Focus for Your Life

Much of diabetes care revolves around food. Your meal plan probably has you eat a certain number of calories, divided among the various Exchanges in a certain way, at certain times each day, every day. When you're trying to lose weight, that focus on food may get stronger. You dread getting hungry; you worry about cravings; you monitor every bite. You may feel you can never just relax and forget about food.

To make matters worse, some women put themselves last in their own lives. They do everything they can to fulfill their children's and husband's

SPOTLIGHT ON RESEARCH
Losing for Yourself Not Others

A report in the *Journal of Personality and Social Psychology* in 1996 looked at whether people's reasons for losing weight affected their success. The researchers gave psychological tests to "severely obese" (their body mass indexes ranged from 31 to 69) people before, during, and after they went on a very-low-calorie diet. At the beginning, 128 people were in the study.

Two years later, during the follow-up, only 52 people were available to be weighed, and only 40 filled out the final tests. The tests were designed to find out the subjects' reasons for joining and staying in the weight-loss program, their beliefs about their control over their own health, and how they felt about the support the weight clinic staff gave them. The researchers then ran statistical tests to see whether the questionnaire results were related to how well people stuck with the program and how much weight they lost.

People who were losing weight for themselves or who thought the clinic staff gave them some control over their progress had better attendance records on average. They also had kept off more weight on average at the follow-up about 2 years later. The researchers concluded that people's reasons for joining a program affect how successful the program will be for them.

goals and dreams. But they deny themselves the same consideration. Eating then becomes one of the few true pleasures they have in life.

If your life revolves around food, try looking for a distraction that's worthwhile and personally fulfilling. Your focus might be people—coaching your kid's Little League team or volunteering at a shelter for homeless people. Or it might be an activity—learning to play the piano or turning your backyard into the neighborhood's most beautiful garden. Whatever you choose, it should be something that gives you joy or peace. It will take up some of the space in your head now crammed with thoughts of calories, fat grams, snack schedules, and dinner menus. You may then be able to break free of constantly thinking about food.

PLAN AHEAD FOR PROBLEMS

No one's path through life is free of obstacles to trip over, forks that veer off into unknown directions, and dark places where you can't see your way. You may not know what problems life has in store for you, but you can be pretty sure you'll face plenty. So it makes sense to plan ahead for them.

Play the "What If?" Game

Imagine everything that could go wrong with your weight-maintenance plan. For example, what if you choose walking as your exercise, and then you get a foot ulcer? What if you visit friends who cook everything in a deep fryer? What if you work an extra 20 hours of overtime a week during your plant's busy season? What if your company often sends you out of town on business? Once you have a list of problems, go through them one by one. Figure out ways to continue to eat right and be active despite them. To come up with even more solutions, invite friends or family members to play this game with you.

Make Constant Course Corrections

When you drive down a straight stretch of highway, you can't aim the steering wheel straight ahead and then assume you'll stay in the center of your lane. The road may veer slightly. Your wheels may be out of alignment. The wind may be gusting. For many reasons, you must constantly adjust the steering wheel to stay on your straight course. You don't consider yourself a driving failure and cancel your trip if you drift across the white line or swerve around an opossum. Likewise, sticking strictly to your meal and exercise plans every day for the rest of your life isn't possible. For many reasons, you must constantly make adjustments to stay on your course to health. You're not a failure if you get the flu and miss a week of exercise or if you sample one of everything at your church's dessert social. Rather, you should note where you are in both body weight and glucose control and correct your course to head in the right direction again.

Rehearse Your Behavior

Play out scenes in your head in which you're tempted to veer from your food plan or skip exercising. You can then practice responses until they feel natural. For example, you can practice saying a simple "No, thank you" over and over to someone who pressures you to eat something you don't want.

By planning ahead, you will be ready to meet whatever challenges life throws at you.

The Skinny on Chapter

19

- ▶ In research studies, people often lose weight for a while. Then weight loss stops, and they start regaining pounds.

- ▶ A body that burns more calories than it takes in loses weight. A body that takes in more calories than it burns puts on weight.

- ▶ Smaller bodies need fewer calories than bigger bodies.

- ▶ Many studies show that exercise slows or prevents weight regain.

- ▶ Hillel pointed out that to have a rich life, a person should have self-respect without being self-centered. These traits are vital in maintaining weight loss as well.

- ▶ Treating yourself with respect and kindness will help you feel you deserve good things in your life.

- ▶ Just as with a stubborn donkey, rewards will help you change your habits.

- ▶ Problems are going to come up in your life. So it makes sense to plan ahead for them.

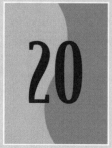

Why Relapses Occur— and What to Do

Human biology and psychology both predict you'll have lapses. But there are ways to triumph in the end.

Some people think relapsing is like being pregnant. Just as you can't be just a little pregnant, these people believe you can't relapse just a little. So if they slip up and fall short of a goal, they assume the battle's over—and they lost.

Other people believe in the "practice makes perfect" model of relapse. If they make a mistake, they try again. They figure they'll know better next time and—maybe—will finally get it right.

Guess which kind of people do better at changing their habits?

Theories and models are useful ways of organizing thoughts and making decisions. So it pays to have good mental models. In this chapter and Chapter 21, you'll learn how psychologists view acquiring good habits and relapsing. These models are important because, as you've seen many times in this book, people tend to regain the weight they lose. This chapter will show that relapsing is normal. You'll learn about the biological pressures to return to your previous weight and the psychological pressures to indulge in behaviors you know aren't good for you. You'll also learn ways to know when you're in danger of relapsing and how to handle these situations. It is possible to prevent weight regain.

WHAT HAPPENS WHEN YOU LOSE WEIGHT

Your body changes when you lose weight. For example, it becomes a bit more fuel efficient. It's no wonder that after losing weight, you can't go back to eating as much food as you used to. Your new, trimmer body just doesn't need as many calories to maintain it as your old, bulkier body did, for several reasons:

- You have reduced the mass that burns calories.

- You have increased your body's efficiency at burning calories.

- Losing weight may trigger your body to turn on emergency energy-conservation measures.

Researchers suspect that after losing weight, people burn less energy when they are at rest, burn less energy after a meal, or burn fat less readily. Any of these ideas, if true, could help explain a strange phenomenon: To stay at a certain weight, say, 200 pounds, people who've lost weight seem to need to eat fewer calories than people who've been that weight all along. Researchers are still trying to figure which of these ideas are right and how big an effect they have. But studies do suggest that the body monitors its weight and adjusts its energy use to regain lost weight or lose gained weight. (See the box "Spotlight on Research: Weight Loss Spurs Metabolism Changes.")

YOUR BODY WANTS TO BE A CERTAIN SIZE AND SHAPE

You've just seen that your body may be reluctant to give up its fat, even if you have more fat than is healthy. But there's more to the story of why it's hard to keep weight off. In some ways, at the time you were born, you were already predisposed to end up a certain size and shape. But this is not to say you can't influence your size and shape—of course you can, as you've seen throughout this book.

Twins and Adoptees

Scientists who want to study the effects of heredity on traits sometimes study twins and adopted people.

SPOTLIGHT ON RESEARCH
Weight Loss Spurs Metabolism Changes

A study in *Metabolism* in 1996 found that losing weight affects people's metabolism. The subjects were 20 people between 55 and 70. All had body mass indexes greater than 32. They ate a reduced-calorie diet for 11 weeks, with about 25% of their calories as fat, 60% as carbohydrate, and 15% as protein.

After 11 weeks, the volunteers had lost an average of 20 pounds. They then spent a couple of days at the research center going through tests. The researchers compared these test results with results from before the weight-loss program. They found that losing weight had several effects on the subjects' metabolism:

- Volunteers burned on average about 15% fewer calories when they were at rest. This is a greater decrease than the researchers expected based on the decrease in body size alone.

- Losing weight did not affect the proportion of fat calories burned when at rest.

- Losing weight did not affect how many extra calories were burned after eating. (Eating causes the body to rev up temporarily.)

- The weight loss did affect what kind of calories were burned. Before weight loss, 38% of the calories burned in the 5 hours after a meal came from fat. After weight loss, only 26% did.

The researchers concluded that losing weight does indeed seem to affect metabolism and that these changes may be one reason why people tend to regain lost weight. Their results suggest that for every kilogram (2.2 pounds) a person loses, he or she burns 2 fewer grams of fat each day. By this rule of thumb, a person who lost 22 pounds would need to cut back on fat intake by 20 grams a day.

Twins allow scientists to tease apart the effects of genes and environment. Identical twins share the same genes. So differences between them cannot be due to inherited factors. Differences must be due to something else. For example, perhaps one got more nourishment in the womb than the other, or one was exposed to a virus the other avoided.

The other kind of twin is fraternal twins. Unlike identical twins, they do not share the same set of genes. Their genes are no more (and no less) alike than those of other pairs of children of the same parents. Differences between fraternal twins can be caused by differences in their life experiences, just as with identical twins. But differences can also be caused by genetic differences. So when a trait differs for genetic reasons, fraternal twins will be less alike than identical twins.

Adoptees are useful in genetic studies for similar reasons. Adoptees resemble their biological families in traits that depend heavily on genes. They resemble their adopted families in traits that depend on living conditions and other external factors.

Studies of adoptees and twins in general have revealed that genetic inheritance is a big influence on people's relative thinness or fatness. (See, for example, the box "Spotlight on Research: Studies in Scandinavia.") But it is not the complete story. Identical twins tend to be similar, but not identical, in body mass index (BMI).

One important thing to keep in mind when you read that a trait has a "high heritability" is that heritability is not an absolute measurement like inches and minutes. Rather, heritability is a relative measurement. It tells you what part of the differences in a trait in a certain group of people cannot be explained by differences in their environments. Just as you would weigh less on the Moon than you do on Earth, even though your body mass is the same, a trait's heritability varies from environment to environment even when the genes remain the same.

Often in studies that show a high genetic component, the twins and adoptees are living in industrialized countries with high standards of living. The habits and home lives of the various families are likely not wildly different. So it's not surprising that most of the differences in BMI among the subjects can be explained by their genes. If the twins or adoptees had lived in a variety of countries and climates and eaten a variety of diets, their environments would have had a bigger effect on their BMIs. So genes would have played a relatively smaller role than in these studies. (If you have trouble understanding why, pretend one identical twin grew up among the Eskimos eating a calorie-dense, meat-rich diet, and the other twin grew up near the equator in a poor country that often suffered famines. Their genes would still be the same. But the differences in their climates and diets would lead to greater differences in their sizes than if both had grown up in Sweden.)

Born to Be Well Insulated

The twin studies and adoptee studies clearly show that inherited factors play big roles in your shape. What are these factors? Scientists do not know for sure, but they have some guesses.

SPOTLIGHT ON RESEARCH
Studies in Scandinavia

The Swedish Adoption/Twin Study of Aging, reported in the *New England Journal of Medicine* in 1990, looked at the influence of genes on BMI. The subjects were 673 pairs of twins in Sweden. Of these twin pairs, 247 were identical twins. Ninety-three pairs were raised apart, and 154 pairs were raised together. Of the fraternal twins, 218 pairs were raised separately, and 208 pairs were raised together. In 1984, the researchers sent questionnaires to the twins and asked for their heights and weights. At that time, the twins ranged in age from the mid-20s to over 80, with an average age of 59.

The researchers ran several statistical tests on the weight and height information to tease apart the effects of genes and rearing environment. Identical twins were quite similar in BMI. Whether they grew up separately or together had little effect. Fraternal twins were much less similar in BMI. In general, male twins were somewhat more alike than female twins. These results show that people's genes had a much bigger effect on their BMI than did their home environment as children.

SPOTLIGHT ON RESEARCH *Continued*

A series of studies in several journals looked at adoptees in Denmark. In Denmark, 5,455 people were adopted by nonrelatives between 1924 and 1947. In the Danish Adoption Study, researchers tracked down as many adoptees as they could and asked them for their height, current weight, and maximum weight. The researchers then collected similar information from the adoptees' biological parents, adoptive parents, biological brothers and sisters, and adoptive brothers and sisters. The researchers were also able to obtain childhood weights and heights for most people who went to schools near Copenhagen.

In the end, the researchers had enough information about several hundred adoptees to include them in statistical analyses. They compared childhood and adult BMIs of the adoptees with the BMIs of both biological and adoptive relatives. The adoptees resembled their adoptive parents, brothers, and sisters slightly in childhood, but not at all as adults. Instead, their BMIs were much more like those of their biological relatives. This similarity developed early. By age 7, children already resembled their biological relatives in BMI. This study, too, shows that genetic inheritance has a strong influence on your shape.

The Thrifty Gene. You met the thrifty gene theory in Chapter 1, and it has come up several times since. Some groups of people, such as Hawaiian natives and American Indians, are at very high risk of obesity and diabetes. These peoples may be especially good at conserving calories—a useful trait during famines, but not so great when food is abundant. Whether this theory is true or not, scientists do know that people vary in how much weight they put on when they eat too much.

Obesity Genes. Chapter 15 briefly mentioned some genes in rats and mice that make them fat. Scientists are just now starting to find genes that cause obesity in humans.

Metabolic Rate. Some people just seem to burn calories more slowly than other people. These differences among people may start early. Researchers have found differences among children, even young babies. A slow metabolism may eventually lead to weight gain in some people.

Natural Activity Level. People vary a lot in how active they are by nature. Some are fidgety; some are still. Some people like sports and moving around; other people prefer quiet pursuits. It's possible that innate differences in activity levels might affect people's weight.

Ratio of Nutrients Burned. There's some evidence that a tendency to burn more fats or more carbohydrates than usual may be inherited.

Climates Your Ancestors Lived In. Body shapes vary quite a bit from climate to climate. Anthropologists have studied these variations for decades and have found they are not random. Rather, bodies are bigger in colder climates, and extremities (ears, noses, arms, legs) are longer in hotter climates. These trends mean that peoples of cold climates tend to have a relatively small surface area (that is, be bulky for their height), which conserves heat. In contrast, peoples of hot climates tend to have a relatively large surface area. This linear shape allows heat to disperse. The effect of climate on shape is partly environmental and partly genetic—that is, anthropologists have found that both the climate you grew up in and the climate your ancestors lived in affect your shape. So if you are shaped more like a ball than a stick, maybe you can blame the weather!

Food Preferences. As you learned in Chapter 9, the ability to taste certain bitter flavors is inherited, and this trait also makes spicy foods taste hotter and sweet foods taste sweeter. Whether other genes exist for food likes and dislikes is not known. But if they do, they might affect weight by influencing what foods you choose to eat.

Keep in mind that inherited differences give you a nudge toward one shape or another. They do not doom you to a life with an unhealthy body shape. Genes act in partnership with the environment in which they find themselves. You can choose to exercise to build muscle and burn fat. You can choose to eat moderate amounts of healthful foods to counteract a tendency to put on weight.

THE PSYCHOLOGICAL SIDE

You now know some biological reasons why keeping weight off can be a fight. But there are plenty of psychological reasons for relapse. Here are a few reasons why people indulge in unhealthful behaviors and have trouble giving them up:

- To fit in: "All my friends smoke."

- To relax: "After a hard day at work, watching TV and having a beer helps me unwind."

- To rebel against authority: "I don't think the government should be telling me how many vegetables to eat."

- To feel loved: "Making my grandmother's special chocolate torte reminds me of when I was little."

- To avoid unpleasantness: "I can't find any exercise I enjoy."

Although psychologists debate the exact number and nature of the psychological forces underlying human behavior, it's clear that the human psyche does require certain things. In 1938, psychologist Henry Murray proposed that humans have 20 basic psychological needs. The reasons above are examples of five. Some other basic needs, according to Murray, are to accomplish hard things, to protect oneself against criticism and other attacks, to avoid embarrassment, to have a sexual relationship, to avoid pain, and to control one's own environment.

How many basic needs can one chocolate bar meet? Several, if you're a chocoholic. It's easy to let food be your friend, your mother, or your lover. It's sometimes harder to find people to nurture you or love you.

WEIGHT CYCLING

As you've learned, it's not only common but normal for your body to try to regain the weight you lose. And, human nature being what it is, it's also common for people to return to ingrained old habits instead of sticking with new, healthful ones. As a result, many people who successfully take off extra pounds later bounce back up to their previous weight. So they start a new weight-loss program and lose the weight again. For some of them, the pounds come back yet another time.

This constant cycle of losing, regaining, losing, and regaining is called weight cycling or "yo-yo dieting." A few years ago, scientists began to study whether weight cycling might have harmful effects on the body.

Theories About Weight Cycling

The idea that weight cycling might be bad for you started when doctors observed that people who had a long history of dieting seemed to have extra trouble taking off weight. Now, this idea may remind you of the children's riddle, "Why do you always find something in the last place you look for it?" (The answer, in case you don't remember, is "Because you stop looking once you find it!") Likewise, people stop trying to lose weight once they no longer need to. So it makes sense that the only people who keep trying and trying to lose weight are those who have not yet been successful at it.

But to some scientists, these observations suggested that another factor might also be at work. Perhaps dieting changed the body in some way so that it became resistant to future dieting.

Since the mid-1980s, researchers have studied the effects of weight cycling. Some theories about weight cycling that you may have read or heard about are:

- People with a history of weight cycling may lose weight at a slower rate or have more trouble keeping it off.

- Weight cycling may increase the amount of fat people have.

- Weight cycling may lower the amount of energy people burn when they are at rest.

- People with a history of weight cycling may have trouble burning body fat.

- Weight cycling may increase blood pressure, blood fats, and other risk factors for heart disease.

- Weight cycling may change people's tastes so that they eat more fat.

- Weight cycling may make certain psychological problems (binge eating or depression) more likely.

Some of these theories have disturbing implications. If weight cycling increased people's fat content or heart disease risk factors, for example, then trying to lose weight would not just be futile. It might also be riskier than staying overweight in the first place!

A Government Report on Weight Cycling

In 1994, the National Task Force on the Prevention and Treatment of Obesity reviewed studies of weight cycling. In most of these studies, the task force concluded that weight cycling:

- Did **not** influence the percentage of fat on the body.

- Did **not** cause fat to shift to less-healthy locations such as the abdomen.

- Did **not** lower the rate at which calories were burned.

- Did **not** predict the success or failure of later weight-loss efforts.

- Did **not** increase fat intake or the desire to eat fat.

- Did **not** worsen blood pressure, glucose or insulin levels, blood fat levels, or other measures associated with the risk of heart disease.

The task force concluded that because the risks of being obese are so clear and the risks of weight cycling are still hazy, people who need to lose weight should try to do so.

But the task force also said that more research on weight cycling is needed. Based on the evidence so far, for instance, it could conclude next to nothing about whether weight cycling causes any psychological harm.

Weight Cycling and Diabetes

Although some scientists studying weight cycling have measured glucose and insulin levels, few studies have focused on people with diabetes. A study in *Health Psychology* in 1990 was an exception. This study looked at medical records of 327 male veterans with type 2 diabetes. The records spanned an average of 3 1/2 years.

The researchers found that about a fifth of the men stayed at a roughly constant weight. They did not gain or lose more than 10% of their starting weight at any time during the study. Some other men gained or lost more than 10% of their weight and stayed there. The rest of the men—about two-thirds of the subjects—weight cycled. At the end of the study, they were within 10% of their starting weight, even though they had gained or lost more than 10% some time in between.

When the researchers compared men who didn't cycle with men who lost and then regained weight and with men who gained and then lost weight, they could find no effect of cycling on diabetes control. All three groups of men had similar fasting glucose and HbA_{1c} (glycated hemoglobin, a measure of long-term glucose control) levels. On average, men in the three groups were taking similar doses of diabetes drugs. In this study, at least, weight cycling had no bad effects on diabetes.

LAPSES AND RELAPSES

Because people often use "relapse" to mean a slip-up, this book does, too. But some psychologists now distinguish between "lapses" and "relapses." A relapse is when you give up on healthful new habits and return to old habits.

In contrast, a lapse occurs when you briefly give in to an old habit. For example, a person under stress may smoke her first cigarette in 5 years or binge on a carton of ice cream. Lapses aren't failures. They are normal events for people who are changing their behavior.

Making a distinction between lapses and relapses gives you more choices. Remember the "pregnancy" and "practice makes perfect" models that opened this chapter? People who subscribed to the "practice makes perfect" model believed in the distinction between lapses and relapses. So they did not despair over minor errors; they got right back on track.

Although lapses can lead to relapses, they don't have to, as the rest of this chapter and Chapter 21 will show you.

RELAPSE-PROOFING YOURSELF

Just as an uneven, potholed road makes it hard to keep control of your car or bike, the bumpy spots of life are the riskiest times for relapse. These may be times that you are sad or angry or nervous. They may be times when you're sick or tired. They may be when you're not getting along with a spouse, friend, or boss.

Even when life is relatively smooth or going well, you may encounter a risky time for relapse. Some people relapse during times of happiness (parties, vacations). Some people are struck by temptations.

According to the Relapse Prevention Model, preventing relapse has three crucial steps:

UP AND DOWN, UP AND DOWN

Roger Esfahani tried every diet there was. In high school, when he weighed more than 300 pounds, he went on a 500-calorie-a-day diet. Even so, he ballooned to nearly 400 pounds in college and then was diagnosed with type 2 diabetes. "In the first couple years of being treated, I went from 400 back down to 300," says Esfahani. He then tried to lose more weight, without much success. "I would yo-yo between 300 and 250 or 270 for the next 8 to 10 years."

He tried commercial nonclinical weight-loss programs, some of them several times. On one program, he lost about 30 pounds. "But as soon as I stopped it, I gained all the weight back," he says.

Susan Lapin has also ridden the weight roller coaster. "I went up to over 200 pounds in high school," she says. But when she went away to college, she started losing weight. "When I graduated from college, I was about 145. And I lived at home for a year and gained 40 pounds." She then left home for good and got her weight back down.

Lapin stayed between 150 and 160 for several years. Then she dieted down to about 145 and got married. Her weight went up and down and then crept up to 185. Two pregnancies and postpartum depression boosted her further. "When my second child was born, I gained about 80 pounds in 6 months," Lapin says. "And I would cry myself to sleep every night because I couldn't stop eating." (In Chapter 21, you'll learn the happy ending to Lapin's story.)

- First, you need to figure out which situations put **you** at risk.

- Second, you must work out possible ways to deal with these times of greatest risk.

- Third, you must accept that lapses are expected. Lapses reveal flaws in the coping methods you've developed. Lapses don't have to turn into relapses.

Risky Situations

In a study in the *Journal of The American Dietetic Association* in 1994, researchers interviewed 12 adults with type 1 diabetes and 14 adults with type 2 diabetes and found that there were 12 kinds of situations in which they had a hard time sticking to a meal plan:

- Negative emotions. You get passed over for a promotion. Or your car breaks down, and you can't afford to get it fixed.

- Resisting temptation. You go to play cards with your friends, and the host puts out bowls of chips, dips, nuts, and pork rinds. Or you have a craving for french fries that won't go away.

- Eating out. You go to an all-you-can-eat buffet. Or you go to a classic French restaurant where rich sauces adorn the specialties.

- Feeling deprived. You look at the people waiting in line at a bakery and feel left out. Or it's your birthday, and having only one piece of cake just doesn't feel like a celebration.

- Time pressure. Keeping your job depends on working double shifts at some times of the year. Or taking care of your house and four kids devours so much time that you get only 4 hours of sleep a night.

- Tempted to relapse. You're tired of measuring portions and feel like giving up. Or you're bored with the 10 healthy recipes you know how to make.

- Planning. You often have to work late without warning. Or your children's soccer practices, trumpet lessons, and dance classes play havoc with your dinner schedule.

- Competing priorities. Caring for an aging mother with Alzheimer's may consume your every waking minute. Or you're head of the synagogue's committee on building an addition, and you need to meet with the zoning board, interview architects and contractors, and fill out piles of paperwork.

- Social events. Your family has a Christmas Eve tradition of sharing fancy desserts. Or for years, your circle of friends has met once a month at a barbecue place.

- Family support. Your husband doesn't want you to lose weight because he's afraid another man will then steal you away. Or your children refuse to eat anything green unless it got that way with the help of FD & C Green Dye No. 3.

- Food refusal. A friend whose feelings are easily hurt offers you a huge piece of her special fruitcake. Or you go to a winter party, and the host makes each guest a fancy hot chocolate topped with fluffy mounds of whipped cream.

- Friends' support. Your best friend has her own ideas about what people with diabetes should eat, and she criticizes every food choice you make. Or a friend who weighs more than you constantly tells you your weight is fine.

Although these risky situations are specifically for sticking with a food plan, many apply to sticking with an exercise plan as well.

When Are You at Risk? And What Will You Do About It?

You've now seen examples of common events and emotions that put people at risk of relapse. To stay on track, adapt the Relapse Prevention Model to your life.

Your Personal Risk Profile. First, go through the list of 12 risky situations. Try to think of ways each might crop up in your own life. Also think about the times you've lost weight before and then regained, or started an exercise program and then quit, or made a good effort to follow your diabetes meal plan and then gave up. What happened? What were your feelings then (for example, were you lonely or frustrated or angry)? Do your relapses have anything in common?

Some people have trigger foods—foods that they can't stop eating once they start. Do you know what yours are?

Think as well about the times when you were able to stick with new habits. How did you motivate yourself? Which behaviors were hard, and which were easy? What do your successes have in common?

SPOTLIGHT ON RESEARCH
Having a Plan Helps Prevent Relapse

A 1994 *Health Psychology* article shows the importance of having a variety of coping strategies. In this study, the subjects were 29 young women who had just joined a health club. They listened to brief descriptions of 10 situations in which sticking to an exercise plan would be hard. Each subject then said how she would get herself to exercise as planned. The subjects also took a test that measured motivation, and they gave some history of their previous exercise attempts.

Fourteen weeks later, the researchers looked at how often the subjects had managed to get to the health club. The researchers defined a lapse as 1 week of no exercise and a relapse as 3 weeks in a row of no exercise.

In just 14 weeks, 19 (66%) of the women had at least one lapse, and 12 had a relapse. Relapsers gave boredom, lack of time, laziness, vacation, and illness as reasons for relapsing.

The researchers compared the 12 relapsers with the 17 women who did not relapse (although some of them did have lapses). Relapsers were three times as likely to have quit an exercise program in the past. Their motivation scores were lower. They also had come up with far fewer coping strategies for the 10 exercise problems. The researchers concluded that having few plans for staying on track during risky times made relapse more likely.

Your Personal Plan to Stay on Track. Second, come up with ways to stick to your new habits in the times you are at risk of relapse. (See the box "Spotlight on Research: Having a Plan Helps Prevent Relapse.") Ways to do this include:

- Brainstorming (the "What If?" game of Chapter 19). Don't censor your thoughts at first. Just write down as many possible solutions as you can, no matter how silly they are. When you look at your list later, you may find several usable ideas.

- Practicing situations in your head ("Rehearse your behavior" in Chapter 19). You can work out kinks in your ideas or plans before risky situations occur in real life.

- Asking friends who've slimmed down or begun exercise programs how they handled lapses. Their methods may work for you.

- Talking to your dietitian. It's his or her job to help you find practical ways to work healthful eating habits into your life.

- Considering a visit with a mental health professional if you often feel lonely or deprived or sad or stressed out. If you learn to deal with these feelings, they will be less likely to trip you up.

Lapses Happen; Be Alert for Them. Third, now you know when you are most at risk of relapse and what you intend to do to fight it. You now need an early-warning system. One useful method is to review your progress each morning and evening. At that time, you can think about what stresses and problems you are facing and what effect they might have on your healthful-living efforts. If you need to, you can also choose how to respond to a stress and put your plan into action.

Another method is to keep a journal or chart of your efforts and successes. You then have an objective record that will show you clearly when you are starting to slip up. You can then take steps to halt the reversal. For example, if you are tracking weight and you see that you are starting to gain instead of lose, then you can limit your calories more strictly and put more effort into exercising. For examples of charts, see Chapter 6.

It's Your Choice

There are many biological pressures on your body to be a certain size and shape. But you can choose to eat right and exercise so that your body is as healthy as possible. There are many psychological needs that overeating and returning to old habits can fill. But you can choose to find other ways to satisfy those needs. Lapses are normal events for people who are changing their lives. But you can still reduce how often they occur by planning ahead and keeping an eye out for risky times. You have plenty of choices.

The Skinny on Chapter

20

▶ After weight loss, your body tries to conserve energy by burning fewer calories.

▶ To learn the effects of heredity on body shape and size, scientists study twins and adoptees.

▶ When environment is important in a trait, unrelated people who live together will be similar.

▶ When genes are important in a trait, closely related people who live apart will be similar, and identical twins will be more alike than fraternal twins.

▶ Inborn differences in food preferences, activity levels, metabolic rates, and ratios of nutrients burned may help explain why particular individuals stay slim or get fat.

▶ Groups of people may differ in their tendency to put on weight because of differences in their ancestral environments—for example, whether their distant ancestors were often subject to food shortages and whether their ancestors needed to conserve heat in a cold climate or disperse heat in a hot climate.

▶ In addition to physical needs such as food and shelter, people have psychological needs. These include the need to avoid injury and the need to feel loved.

▶ Many unhealthful habits are hard to break because they fill psychological needs.

The Skinny on Chapter 20
Continued

▶ Weight cycling, or yo-yo dieting, is a pattern of losing weight and regaining it over and over.

▶ Early studies suggested that weight cycling might hinder later weight-loss efforts, increase the risk of heart and blood vessel diseases, or cause mental anguish.

▶ Fears about weight cycling seem unfounded, at least given the results of studies so far.

▶ A lapse is when a person strays briefly from good habits.

▶ A relapse occurs when a person abandons good habits and returns to unhealthful habits.

▶ The three steps of relapse prevention are to identify risky situations, to plan responses to stay on track during these situations, and to accept that lapses happen to everyone and can help show where planned responses are not up to snuff.

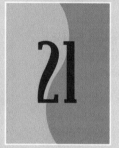

CHAPTER

21

Worms do it; frogs
do it; dogs do it.
All can learn new
behaviors—and so
can you.

How Habits Change

In the final few years of the 1800s, a scientist studying digestion discovered some weird ways to make dogs slobber. Ivan Pavlov gave his dog subjects powdered meat to whet their appetites and stimulate saliva, which he then collected. But after awhile, he found that the dogs were salivating even before they were fed. Just looking at their food made them drool. So did hearing the footsteps of the experimenter bringing in the meat powder. Pavlov tried ringing a bell at mealtime. After awhile, the dogs salivated when they heard a bell. By a similar method, Pavlov taught them to salivate when they saw a drawing of a circle or heard the ticking of a metronome.

Teaching dogs to slobber may not seem particularly useful. But these experiments opened scientists' eyes to how animals learn behaviors. In the century since, psychologists have greatly expanded our knowledge of learning. Today, psychologists can use the basic principles of learning to train all sorts of creatures, even very simple ones with hardly any brain at all, to do all sorts of things. These same principles work to change human behavior as well.

In this chapter, you'll learn about some approaches to acquiring good habits. You'll also see, from two points of view, how people who have lost weight and prevented regain managed to do it. These people are proof that it is possible to lose weight for good.

HOW HABITS FORM

Habits are a way the brain automates actions it does over and over. Habits save time and effort. When a child suddenly darts in front of your car, you slam on the brakes and veer away. You don't consciously run through a list of possible outcomes and calculate their probabilities, produce a list of options, and choose the course of action with the best cost-benefit ratio. You don't consciously pull your right foot from the gas pedal and feel around on the floor for the brake. You already have routines—habits—for recognizing dangerous driving situations and reacting. You already have habits that make the steering wheel and brake pedal seem parts of your body. Driving was quite different when you were a teen. You had to think about what to do in each situation. Even so, you may still have rammed your parents' garage door or driven into a ditch or two.

Psychologists recognize two main types of learning. One is called classic conditioning. When two things occur together, the mind learns to link them. Either can trigger a response that only one triggered before. Pavlov's dogs first learned to associate footsteps with food because the experimenter came in at mealtimes. Later, footsteps made them salivate even if they received no food. In this same way, people may develop a craving to eat while watching TV or at a party, even when they're not hungry.

A second type of learning is operant conditioning. When something pleasant accompanies or follows an action, you learn to do it more often. When something unpleasant occurs instead, you learn to avoid doing it. Take weighing yourself. You may get on the scale every morning when you're losing weight because you expect good news. But you avoid the scale when you're regaining because you expect to be disappointed.

Habits are comforting, familiar, natural. Changing habits disrupts your life. Cats are a good example of a creature bound by habit. A new brand of cat litter in their box or suddenly getting dinner after sunset after daylight saving time ends is a major cat crisis. Humans are pretty adaptable. But like cats, we still find it unpleasant to have our routines turned upside down. As a result, just as operant conditioning would predict, people resist learning new habits.

Luckily, the two forms of conditioning that helped you acquire bad habits in the first place can help you learn new, good habits now.

STAGES OF CHANGE

Many health professionals use the so-called Stages-of-Change Model of James Prochaska to describe how people give up bad habits for good ones. The model seems to fit many kinds of unhealthy behaviors: eating too much fat, not exercising, smoking, using drugs, and not getting mammograms, among others. No matter what the habit, people seem to pass through the same five stages while changing it.

- The first stage is called the precontemplation stage. At this stage, people have no intention of changing. The cons of changing outweigh the pros for them. They may not believe that they even have a problem.

- The second stage is contemplation. People at this stage do see that they have a problem. They are thinking about making a change within the next 6 months. But they have not yet made up their minds for sure.

- The third stage is preparation. People in this stage have decided to make a change within the next month. But they have not yet gotten started.

- The fourth stage is action. In this stage, people stop thinking about changing and actually do it.

- The fifth stage is maintenance. This stage starts when a person has made the change and stuck with it for at least 6 months. After this length of time, the new behavior no longer seems so hard. It's become a habit.

Moving Through the Stages

It's rare for people to stride through all five stages in order and stay in the maintenance stage for good. Many people stay in precontemplation forever. Some get stuck in contemplation or preparation, always on the verge of changing but never quite getting around to doing it.

Many people spiral. They advance, then go back to an earlier stage, then advance again. For example, someone may decide to quit smoking (preparation stage), then decide that smoking is too enjoyable to give up (precontemplation stage). Later, perhaps when a child gets asthma or when a heart attack strikes, the smoker may enter the contemplation stage again. Or a family may have adopted a low-fat diet (action stage) and stuck to it for 8 months (so entering the maintenance stage). But during a crisis, they may not have the energy or time to cook healthful meals. They may plan to start again when the problem is over (preparation stage).

Using the Stages-of-Change Model in Your Own Life

This model can help you in several ways as you think about healthful habits. First, it reveals change as the personal and unique dance it really is, not as a march in lockstep with everyone else. Forward and back, back and forward, you may cycle through stages awhile before you spend much time in maintenance. This spiraling is normal. It can even be helpful. It gives you a chance to learn from your mistakes so that you'll do better on your next try.

Second, it's useful to know that the first three stages take place mostly in your head. Spending a lot of time weighing the pros and cons is a normal part of deciding to make a change. You shouldn't be frustrated if it takes you awhile to get started on—or get back to—healthful habits. Successful change depends on coming to believe that healthful habits are worth the effort.

Third, researchers have found that people in certain stages are most open to certain kinds of help. If you are moving from precontemplation to contemplation, you can be helped by:

- Consciousness raising: learning about the risks of the unhealthful behavior and the good effects of switching to a more healthful one

- Dramatic relief: letting yourself feel the range of emotions associated with the unhealthful behavior—for example, anger at the thought of giving up a familiar habit, distress over the harm that may befall you if you don't, shock or grief over a friend who died from a heart attack

- Environmental reevaluation: becoming aware of how your unhealthful behavior affects your family, your pets, your home, and your social and work life—for example, are you shortening your children's lives by setting a bad example for them to follow?

As you move into contemplation, another method joins the first three:

- Self-reevaluation: contrasting how you see yourself now as a person who smokes, eats a high-fat diet, is sedentary, or has some other unhealthful behavior with how you'll see yourself when you're a nonsmoker or an active person

After you've moved from contemplation to preparation, you know why a change is a good idea and are preparing yourself to deal with the change. Now, another method may help you move to action:

- Self-liberation: making a decision to change, committing to the change, and believing that you can do it

When you enter the action stage, several new aids come to the forefront. Their help continues during the maintenance stage:

- Reinforcement: praising yourself, giving yourself rewards for each small step, being praised by other people for your change

- Helping relationships: having people to talk to about your change, getting support for your decision

- Counterconditioning: replacing unhealthful choices with healthful ones, such as using skim milk instead of whole milk or going for a walk when you're stressed instead of eating ice cream

- Stimulus control: changing your environment to make healthful habits easier, such as not allowing high-fat foods in your house or avoiding situations in which you overeat

If you can figure out where you are, you can tailor your weight-loss approach to that stage. For example, if you're in contemplation, it may help to learn as much as you can about the dangers of obesity and poor diabetes control and do some soul searching about how you feel about your weight. But if you're in the action stage, it's more useful to collect tips for cutting fat from your diet and finding time to exercise.

BEHAVIORAL MODIFICATION

"Behavioral modification" is a grab bag of techniques for changing behavior. They are based on what psychologists know about the effects of rewards and punishments on behavior. Unlike some psychological methods, which delve into the roots of behavior, behavioral modification focuses on the behavior itself and ignores its causes.

Dog obedience classes offer a good example of behavioral modification. The teacher makes no effort to find out why Rex bites strangers in

WHEN MOTIVATION STRIKES

Sometimes, out of the blue, the will to lose weight joins the desire to. "It's like something comes and sits over your head like a holy flame that allows you to stay on a diet," says Susan Lapin. "All of a sudden you've got the motivation. You don't know where it came from. You don't know how to bring it out again—but it's there."

Once she lost some weight, the benefits motivated her even more. At her heaviest, she was 346 pounds. "When you weigh that much, you're limited in how far you can walk, how long you can stand, what chairs you can sit on, everything. Everything has to be pre-planned," Lapin says. In contrast, after losing 75 pounds, she now feels free and strong. "I can walk more than a mile. I can stand. I can work in my garden." She also enjoys her children's praise.

"If I can get under 200 pounds, I will be a happy lady," she says. To stay on track, she weighs herself every single day and monitors how her clothes are fitting.

the buttocks or sits with his rear paws sticking out in front. Rather, the teacher guides you in using rewards and punishments to get your dog to obey your commands and have good posture while doing so.

Some weight-loss clinics teach behavior-modification methods to their patients. The idea is that people can use these tools to wean themselves from unhealthful behaviors and to acquire good habits. This idea makes a lot of sense. If you can train a dog to stand quietly and ignore the urge to lunge at a passing squirrel, you may be able to train yourself to eat moderately and ignore the urge to lunge at the last brownie on the plate. Many of the ideas you've met already in this book—such as giving yourself a present when you meet a goal (Chapter 19) and making your meal seem more filling (Chapter 10)—are behavior-modification techniques.

Some researchers use a four-step behavior-modification plan to help people change their eating and exercise habits. The steps are simple, and you can follow them at home.

1. Have a clear idea what behavior you want to change. Keeping a diary of everything you eat will show you exactly what you are eating now. It can also be a way to track your progress to healthier habits later.

2. Set short-term goals. For example, you might decide to lose 1 pound this week and to exercise 4 days this week. For this step to work, you need a way to know whether your behavior change is working. Here's where the bathroom scale comes in. It can let you know whether you really have changed your behavior and how effective those changes are.

3. Figure out what triggers a behavior for you, and brainstorm ways to control those triggers. For example, if seeing food around the house makes you want to eat, you might keep foods stored in closed cabinets. If you have trouble resisting food urged on you at parties, you might rehearse saying "no." If you can never remember to exercise, putting your shoes next to the door may help.

4. Change the rewards you get from your habits. Eating high-fat food is fun. So is lying around watching TV. To increase the appeal of more healthful habits, you can reward yourself with money or nonfood treats.

Some studies find that people, including people with diabetes, have an easier time losing weight or keeping weight off if they are taught behavior-modification methods. But other studies find behavioral modification has no effect on weight loss or that the effects soon wear off. More research is needed to fine-tune behavioral modification so that it works more reliably and its effects last longer.

SUCCESSFUL WEIGHT LOSERS, AS SEEN BY RESEARCHERS

It's now clear that being overweight is a long-term problem, not something that can be solved easily once and for all. As a result, scientists have become interested in why some people do better at preventing weight regain than others. Researchers are starting to look at the similarities among people who've successfully lost weight in research studies. They have found that research subjects lose and keep off the most weight when they:

- Exercise

- Take part in long, slow treatment programs rather than ones that cover the material more quickly

- Take part in treatment programs that are very structured, such as those with strict diets

- Take part in treatment programs that include doctors, nurses, dietitians, psychologists, and exercise specialists

- Enroll in a maintenance program or get long-term follow-up care

- Receive support from friends or relatives

These results may not tell the whole story, however. First, some researchers think people who sign up for weight-loss studies are not typical of people who lose weight on their own. Study subjects may be willing to put up with a study's strict rules and lack of personalization because they've been unable to take off weight by their own efforts. Second, these results are based on the researchers' observations of group averages. So they focus on external events that are common to an entire group. They cannot reveal precisely what happened in Mary's life or Joe's thoughts that made a difference.

SUCCESSFUL WEIGHT LOSERS, AS SEEN BY THEMSELVES

Some researchers are starting to ask successful weight losers directly how they did it. These studies provide the first evidence of the methods people find most useful. These methods may help you lose weight and maintain it as well.

A Study of HMO Members

A 1990 *American Journal of Clinical Nutrition* article reported on 108 women in a health-maintenance organization (HMO). Some women had always been at a normal weight, whereas others had been more than 20% overweight at some time. Interviews with the women revealed that those who had lost weight and kept it off ("maintainers") differed in some ways from those who regained weight ("relapsers"). Among these differences:

- Maintainers did not just adopt a set of strategies given them by a doctor or class. Rather, the women devised their own plans to fit the conditions of their lives. These personalized plans tended to include exercising, cutting fat and sugar, and eating more produce. Relapsers tended not to develop their own plans. Instead, they were far more likely to join a group or formal weight-loss program or to follow their doctors' orders.

- Maintainers were twice as likely to exercise as relapsers. Relapsers who did exercise did so less than maintainers.

- Relapsers were more likely to try quick-fix ideas, such as fasting, hypnosis, or drastic diets.

- Maintainers let themselves have their favorite foods and other treats sometimes. Relapsers tended to deny themselves foods they enjoyed. They also felt deprived on their weight-loss plans.

- Relapsers seemed surprised that weight came back when they stopped their weight-loss plan. Maintainers knew they had to stick with their new habits.

- Relapsers averaged three times as many snacks a day. They also tended to eat more candy and chocolate.

- Maintainers coped with problems in their lives by confronting the problems, trying to figure out solutions, talking about their problems, or distracting themselves by exercising, working, or shopping. Relapsers tended to cope with problems by eating, smoking, sleeping, and wishing the problem would go away.

- Relapsers were less likely to have friends or family members they could count on for support.

Of course, some of these factors may merely be markers for what's really going on behind the scenes. Exercising is tied tightly in this study and many others to success in keeping weight off. Is this success due entirely to extra physical activity? Or is it partly due to a personality trait—for example, that people who are good at sticking to exercise also are good at sticking to low-calorie food plans?

Interestingly, women who had always been at a normal weight seemed not to be that way by accident. Rather, they had long had many healthful habits. In many ways, their usual behaviors resembled those of women who were consciously trying to keep lost weight from returning.

The National Weight Control Registry

To study traits of people who successfully lose weight, researchers found 784 adults who had both lost at least 30 pounds and kept at least that much weight off for at least 1 year. The results were reported in the *American Journal of Clinical Nutrition* in 1997.

The 629 women and 155 men filled out several questionnaires that asked many questions about their weight, weight-loss methods, and weight-maintenance methods. Most had become overweight as children, and most had at least one overweight parent. Yet despite this predisposition to overweight, they dropped an average of about 10 1/2 body mass index units.

The researchers found that:

- The subjects had used a wide variety of weight-loss and weight-maintenance methods, suggesting that people do best when they choose a method that fits their own life.

- Almost everyone both cut calories and exercised, rather than focusing on one or the other.

- The subjects exercised quite a bit more than the average American. More than half burned at least 2,000 calories a week.

- They ate much less fat than most Americans, averaging 24% of calories from fat.

- Half continued to count calories and/or fat grams during weight maintenance.

- Half of the people weighed themselves every day. About a quarter stepped on the scales less than once a week.

- Something happened in the lives of three-quarters of the people to make this weight-loss attempt different from all the ones before. Maybe they got a shock when they saw a photograph of themselves, or a new health problem scared them into taking action.

The Bottom Line

Presumably, it's not coincidence that studies find that maintainers share many actions and attitudes. These may be what helped them keep weight off. If so, then to lose weight permanently, you would be wise to:

- Continue following a reduced-calorie meal plan.
- Exercise.
- Use problem-solving approaches to life's problems instead of trying to avoid them.
- Build a support team of family or friends.
- Accept the need to stick to your healthful habits.
- Personalize your weight loss to your own life rather than taking your doctor's or weight-loss clinic's word as the one true path to weight loss.
- Make room in your life for treats and happy times.

People from all different walks of life, who are overweight for all different kinds of reasons, have lost weight successfully. You can, too!

The Skinny on Chapter

- ► The brain automates some actions to save time and effort.

- ► Pavlov's dogs learned to salivate when they heard a bell because the bell rang before they got their food. This kind of learning is classic conditioning.

- ► A dog that receives a bone each time it barks will learn to bark more often. A dog that is scolded each time it barks will learn to bark less often. This kind of learning is operant conditioning.

- ► Habits are pleasant. Changing habits is not.

- ► The Stages-of-Change Model explains change as a process that involves deciding whether change is even a good idea, deciding whether to make a change, actually making the change, and trying to stay with the change.

- ► Behavioral modification is a way of adopting the principles of conditioning to help people make changes more easily and stick with them.

- ► Because fighting overweight is a lifetime commitment, scientists are starting to look at why some people lose weight permanently but others lose and then regain.

- ► Study after study shows that continuing to restrict calorie intake and being active are crucial to keeping weight off.

- ► Treatment programs may help people most when they are very structured, include a variety of health professionals, last a long time, and provide follow-up care.

- ► People are more likely to keep weight off if they exercise, mold their weight-loss effort around their life instead of forcing their life to conform to someone else's ideas, include room for treats in their food plan, confront problems, and have supportive friends or relatives.

- ► People are more like to relapse if they just follow doctor's orders, don't exercise, try get-thin-quick schemes, deny themselves foods they like, snack often, run away from problems, lack a support system, and stop healthy habits after losing weight.

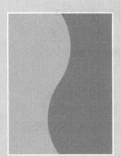

You have what it takes to take weight off.

Afterword: You Can Do It!

You now know a lot about what scientists have learned—and haven't learned—about losing weight. You know that no special talent is required. Neither is willpower beyond the reach of normal humans. You don't need a magic plan either, because there is no one right way to lose weight.

The only hard-and-fast rule is to take in fewer calories than you burn.

Scientists have learned that there are hard ways to achieve this goal, and there are easier ways. This book boils down the mountains of research on weight loss into seven keys. These keys tip you off to what works well and what doesn't. They can help you chart an effective, practical course to a healthier body.

Key 1. Choosing the Right Target Weight Can Make the Difference Between Success and Failure. Each person is unique. So weight goals should be, too. Few people need to get down to a "normal" weight to feel better and be healthier. In fact, for many people, a first goal of losing 5% to 10% is a good one. It's doable and can improve many health problems, including diabetes.

Key 2. The Best Way of Measuring Your Weight-Loss Progress Is by Tracking Your Health (Not Just

Your Weight). Probably, one of your major reasons for losing weight is to help your diabetes. Tracking glucose gives you vital information about how you're doing. So can monitoring improvements in other aspects of your health, such as blood pressure.

Key 3. A Healthful, Low-Calorie Diet Is the Only Good Way to Take Off Pounds. Weight loss is fastest and easiest when people make cutting calories the central feature of a weight-loss plan. The Food Guide Pyramid points the way to eating habits that help you control your diabetes and lose weight. The Pyramid may seem complex, but almost all its advice can be distilled into three sentences:

- There are no "bad" or "evil" foods.

- Plant foods (grains, fruits, vegetables, and beans) should make up most of your diet.

- Foods that have few nutrients or that are high in fat or sugar are best as accents to meals, not as the focus.

Key 4. An Active Lifestyle Helps Lost Pounds Stay Lost. Exercise counteracts the body's tendency to regain weight and slashes your risk of many diseases. Any activity that burns calories and gets you moving is good. And it's okay to choose fun things such as dancing or gardening or walking in the mall. Having fun makes sticking with an active lifestyle easier.

Key 5. If You Have a Lot of Weight to Lose, Modern Medicine Has Some Extra Help to Offer. Doctors offer other weight-loss options, including very-low-calorie diets, weight-loss drugs, and stomach surgeries. These are not for everyone. They have side effects and can be dangerous. But for some people, these aids can tip the scales in their favor.

Key 6. Your Weight-Loss Program Must Coordinate With Your Diabetes Care. Diabetes itself can affect your weight. So can its treatments. If you understand their effects, weight loss will go more smoothly.

Key 7. Permanent Weight Loss Requires That You Change Your Lifestyle for Good. Last, but certainly not least, is the key to preventing weight regain. Adopting new habits is vital to staying at a new, thinner weight. People who return to their previous lifestyle return as well to their previous weight.

Do you have what it takes? Certainly!

It doesn't matter if you haven't succeeded before. Plenty of people have to try many times before finally succeeding.

It also doesn't matter if you're not good at doing without life's pleasures. Few people **could** keep up a joyless life for long. But trying new foods and activities can be exciting. And a full, vibrant life helps your weight-loss efforts by keeping you busy and active.

It doesn't even matter if you're 200 pounds overweight. You can still become healthier and happier. You don't need to get down to an ideal weight before you start feeling better. Good effects should start kicking in after you've lost just 10 or 15 pounds. And your glucose level may drop even sooner.

You can do it!

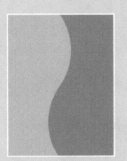

Resources

BOOKS/PAMPHLETS/COOKBOOKS

Dietary Guidelines for Americans

The *Dietary Guidelines for Americans* discuss in very simple language what constitutes a healthy weight and a healthful diet. The American Diabetes Association says these guidelines are suitable for people with diabetes. To get a copy of the guidelines, send your name and address and a check for 50¢ to:

> Consumer Information Center
> Department 378-C
> Pueblo, CO 81009

Or you can read a text-only version (that is, it lacks a Food Guide Pyramid, the graph of suggested weights, and other useful pictures) on the World Wide Web at http://www.pueblo.gsa.gov/cic_text/fd&nut/dietary.txt.

Learning About Diabetes

The American Diabetes Association can help you learn more about diabetes. It publishes many books on a variety of topics related to diabetes. Books about different types of diabetes include:

- *The Take-Charge Guide to Type I Diabetes*

- *Type 2 Diabetes: Your Healthy Living Guide*

- *Gestational Diabetes: What to Expect*

A book that covers many facets of type 1, type 2, and gestational diabetes is:

- *American Diabetes Association Complete Guide to Diabetes*

You can also access brochures about diabetes and a variety of other information online. ADA's World Wide Web site is at http://www. diabetes.org/. In addition, ADA has an area on America Online at keyword AMERICAN DIABETES.

Calculating Nutrition Information

The American Diabetes Association book *The Diabetes Carbohydrate and Fat Gram Guide,* by Lea Ann Holzmeister, lists calorie, carbohydrate, and fat contents for almost anything you could possibly eat. And it fits in a purse.

WINning the Weight-Loss Game

The Weight-Control Information Network (WIN) is a service of the National Institute of Diabetes and Digestive and Kidney Diseases. From WIN you can get a variety of fact sheets and pamphlets related to weight control. These include *Physical Activity and Weight Control, Prescription Medications for the Treatment of Obesity, Understanding Adult Obesity, Very Low-Calorie Diets, Statistics Related to Overweight and Obesity,* and *Weight Cycling.*

You can call the toll-free number 800-946-8098 to leave your name and address to get a sample packet of materials. You can also download some of these from WIN's website at http://www.niddk.nih.gov/Nutrition Docs.html.

Evaluating Weight-Loss Programs

Weighing the Options: Criteria for Evaluating Weight-Management Programs is a book for consumers prepared by the Institute of Medicine and published by the National Academy Press. The book is a rich source of information about losing weight in general and about choosing weight-loss programs in particular. For example, it summarizes the methods, costs, and philosophies of many popular programs. It also has some quizzes to help you decide if you are ready to start a weight-loss program.

This 1995 book is available from the National Academy Press (800-624-6242 or, for people who live near Washington, DC, 202-334-3313). Your local bookstore should be able to order it as well, or your library may have it.

You can also order the book online at http://www.nap.edu/book store/isbn/0309051312.html. The site has an uncorrected proof that you can read on your computer. Be aware, though, that each Web page contains only one scanned text page, so this option is quite slow and costly unless you have a very, very fast and cheap Internet connection.

Cooking for People With Diabetes

The American Diabetes Association publishes more than three dozen cookbooks. Although many low-fat, heart-healthy cookbooks are suitable for people with diabetes, the ADA books list the Exchanges for each recipe. So they make it easy to fit your menu to your diabetes meal plan.
ADA cookbooks include:

- *How to Cook for People with Diabetes*. Reprints of recipes that first appeared in the magazine *Diabetes Forecast*.

- *Flavorful Seasons Cookbook*. Four hundred recipes keyed to the changing temperatures and moods of the four seasons.

- *World-Class Diabetic Cooking*. Low-fat, low-calorie recipes inspired by cuisines around the world.

- *Your Key to Healthy Persian Cooking*. Exotic but comforting food fit for a king.

- *The Healthy HomeStyle Cookbook*. Traditional American fare, lightened up for modern tastes.

- *Diabetic Meals In 30 Minutes—Or Less!* Fast recipes packed with flavor, many suitable for company.

- *Holiday Cookbook.* Tempting, healthy feasts for Thanksgiving, Hanukkah, and Christmas.

Nutrition Information on the Web

The World Wide Web is home to mountains of nutrition information. Here are a few sites where you can learn more about food and nutrition.

- The American Dietetic Association's site contains dozens of Nutrition Fact Sheets. It is at http://www.eatright.org.

- At the American Heart Association's site, you'll find heart-healthy recipes, nutrition information, lists of brochures you can order, and descriptions of American Heart Association cookbooks. It is at http://www.amhrt.org.

- The National Cancer Institute's 5 A Day site has some recipes and many tips for eating more fruits and vegetables. And if you want to advertise your passion for produce, you can order T-shirts and other merchandise with the 5 A Day logo. The 5 A Day site is at http://www. dcpc.nci.nih.gov/5aday/.

- Many government brochures and pamphlets are available online at the Consumer Information Center's site. Most contain just text with no graphics. The two areas of this site with nutrition information are http://www.pueblo.gsa.gov/food.htm and http://www.pueblo.gsa.gov/other/o-food.htm.

- The Minnesota Attorney General's Office compiled a list of nutrition information about fast food. These data are now available at the Fast Food Finder site, where you can look up the calories, fat, sodium, and cholesterol in your favorite fast foods. It is at http://www.olen.com/food/.

- At the Dole Food Company's site, Bobby Banana guides children (and adults) through learning about fruits and vegeta-

bles. The site contains recipes and lots of information on specific kinds of produce. It is at http://www.dole5aday.com.

- Another commercial site worth a look is that of the Calorie
  Control Council (a trade association of companies that make
  or supply low-calorie or low-fat foods). It focuses on artificial
  sweeteners and fat substitutes, but you can also look up the
  number of calories and fat grams in many kinds of food. You
  can find it at http://www.caloriecontrol.org.

ORGANIZATIONS THAT PROVIDE FREE (OR CHEAP) INFORMATION ABOUT FITNESS

Shape Up America! is a national campaign led by former Surgeon General
C. Everett Koop. Its goal is to teach Americans the benefits of a healthy
weight and how to become more active. It has four brochures for the
general public: *99 Tips for Family Fitness Fun, Fitting Fitness In Even When
You're Pressed for Time, On Your Way To Fitness,* and *Eating Smart, Even
When You're Pressed for Time.* You can receive any or all of these by calling the toll-free number 888-U-SHAPE-IT (888-872-7348).

Although it is primarily a professional association for health professionals and scientists, the **American College of Sports Medicine** also
has several brochures for the general public. These include *ACSM
Health/Fitness Facility Consumer Selection Guide, Exercise Lite, Sports
Medicine Umbrella, Play It Safe! A guide to preventing sports-related
injuries in young athletes, Nutrition and Sports Performance: A Guide for
Physically-Active Young People,* and *Staying Fit Over 40.* Your first copy of
each is free.

ACSM also has several low-cost brochures. These include *Achieving
and Maintaining Physical Fitness* ($2), *Alcohol in Sports* ($1), *Weight-Loss
Programs* ($1), *Prevention of Heat Injuries During Running* ($1), and *Youth
Fitness* ($1). (These are 1998 prices.)

To get a free brochure, send a self-addressed, stamped business-size
envelope to ACSM Public Information Department, P.O. Box 1440,
Indianapolis, IN 46206-1440. To get a brochure that costs something,
send a check (but not an envelope) to the same address.

OTHER HEALTH ORGANIZATIONS

The **American Dietetic Association** can refer you to a professional dietitian in your area.

You can contact them at 216 West Jackson Boulevard, Suite 800, Chicago, IL 60606. Their toll-free number is 800-366-1655. See the list of Web sites to contact them online.

The **American Heart Association (AHA)**, like many other organizations, issues guidelines. Their 1996 dietary guidelines contain the most up-to-date information on preventing heart and blood vessel disease. These guidelines mirror the *Dietary Guidelines for Americans* in almost every way, but AHA makes a few extra suggestions.

You can contact AHA at 7272 Greenville Avenue, Dallas, TX 75231. The toll-free number is 800-242-8721. See the list of Web sites above to contact them online.

Index

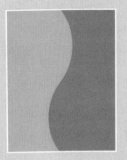

About the Authors

Barbara Caleen Hansen, PhD, is internationally recognized for her work on obesity, diabetes, and aging. She was the first president of the International Association for the Study of Obesity, has served as president of the North American Association for the Study of Obesity and the American Society for Clinical Nutrition, and is a member of the Institute of Medicine of the National Academy of Sciences. Author of numerous articles and book contributions in the fields of weight regulation and diabetes, she is currently Professor of Physiology and Director of the Obesity and Diabetes Research Center at the School of Medicine of the University of Maryland, Baltimore.

Shauna S. Roberts, PhD, is a science writer and editor who specializes in diabetes. She is the Contributing Editor of *The Diabetes Advisor* newsletter, and she often writes for *Diabetes Forecast* magazine. She also wrote many of the American Diabetes Association's patient brochures. Formerly a biological anthropologist, she has long been fascinated by the physical and cultural differences among people. She received her BA from the University of Pennsylvania in Philadelphia and her MA and PhD from Northwestern University in Evanston, Illinois. When not writing, she plays harp, recorders, and harpsichord in early music ensembles. She also enjoys quilting, growing herbs, and making bread.

About the American Diabetes Association

The American Diabetes Association is the nation's leading voluntary health organization supporting diabetes research, information, and advocacy. Founded in 1940, the Association provides services to communities across the country. Its mission is to prevent and cure diabetes and to improve the lives of all people affected by diabetes.

For more than 50 years, the American Diabetes Association has been the leading publisher of comprehensive diabetes information for people with diabetes and the health care professionals who treat them. Its huge library of practical and authoritative books for people with diabetes covers every aspect of self-care—cooking and nutrition, fitness, weight control, medications, complications, emotional issues, and general self-care. The Association also publishes books and medical treatment guides for physicians and other health care professionals.

Membership in the Association is available to health care professionals and people with diabetes and includes subscriptions to one or more of the Association's periodicals. People with diabetes receive *Diabetes Forecast*, the nation's leading health and wellness magazine for people with diabetes. Health care professionals receive one or more of the Association's five scientific and medical journals.

For more information, please call toll-free:

Questions about diabetes: 1-800-DIABETES

Membership, people with diabetes: 1-800-806-7801

Membership, health professionals: 1-800-232-3472

Free catalog of ADA books: 1-800-232-6733

Visit us on the Web: . . . . www.diabetes.org